8/10

# THE SEVEN STEPS TO KEYBOARDING FOR SUCCESS:

## A Comprehensive Guide for All Computer Users

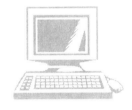

CHARLENE H. GRAFTON

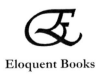

Eloquent Books

Strategic Book Publishing or Eloquent Books
An imprint of Strategic Book Group
P.O.Box 333
Durham, CT 06422


www.StrategicBookGroup.com

ISBN: 978-1-60911-020-8

Printed in the United States of America

*To all Americans who consider themselves a computer user and who work six to eight hours or more each day. Also to those users who (or) to those same users, who are having computer related problems due to long-time use at their workstation. And to those same computer users who want to know the how and why they can improve their productivity with peripheral input devices to use with changes at their PC or laptop workstation.*

# TABLE OF CONTENTS

Acknowledgements . . . . . . . . . . . . . . . . . . . . . . . . . . . . . . . . . . . . . . . . . . ix

**PART ONE:**
**COMPUTER WORKSTATION: WE HAVE A PROBLEM    1**
Introduction . . . . . . . . . . . . . . . . . . . . . . . . . . . . . . . . . . . . . . . . 3

**Chapter One**
Carpal Tunnel Syndrome And Other
Muscle And Tendon Disorders . . . . . . . . . . . . . . . . . . . . . . . . 17

**Chapter Two**
Types Of Treatment . . . . . . . . . . . . . . . . . . . . . . . . . . . . . . . . 27

**PART TWO:**
**CLEAR AND CONVINCING EVIDENCE            31**
**Chapter Three**
Factors To Consider . . . . . . . . . . . . . . . . . . . . . . . . . . . . . . . . 33

**Chapter Four**
Alternative Solutions . . . . . . . . . . . . . . . . . . . . . . . . . . . . . . . 39

**Chapter Five**
Background Information . . . . . . . . . . . . . . . . . . . . . . . . . . . . . 53

**Chapter Six**
Case Histories . . . . . . . . . . . . . . . . . . . . . . . . . . . . . . . . . . . . 63

**PART THREE:**
**FOLLOW THE RIGHT ROAD                      67**
**Chapter Seven**
The Exercises . . . . . . . . . . . . . . . . . . . . . . . . . . . . . . . . . . . . . 69

**Chapter Eight**
Establishing Directionality . . . . . . . . . . . . . . . . . . . . . . . . . . . 83

**PART FOUR:**
**TRAINING THE LEFT HAND FOR**
**COMPUTER USAGE**                                    **99**

**Chapter Nine**
Dexterity Training . . . . . . . . . . . . . . . . . . . . . . . . . . . . . . . 101

**Chapter Ten**
Numerical Data Training . . . . . . . . . . . . . . . . . . . . . . . . . 109

**Chapter Eleven**
Finding Your Target . . . . . . . . . . . . . . . . . . . . . . . . . . . . . 123

**Chapter Twelve**
Mouse Training . . . . . . . . . . . . . . . . . . . . . . . . . . . . . . . . . 131

**PART FIVE:**
**ENDLESS POSSIBILITIES**                              **139**

**Chapter Thirteen**
Brain Organization And Networking . . . . . . . . . . . . . . . . . 141

**Chapter Fourteen**
Musicians And Typists . . . . . . . . . . . . . . . . . . . . . . . . . . . 155

**Chapter Fifteen**
Performance And Individual Differences . . . . . . . . . . . . . . 163

**PART SIX:**
**ONLY YOU CAN MAKE A DIFFERENCE**                     **177**

**Chapter Sixteen**
Hand And Finger Movements . . . . . . . . . . . . . . . . . . . . . . 179

**Chapter Seventeen**
All About Learning. . . . . . . . . . . . . . . . . . . . . . . . . . . . . . 189

**Chapter Eighteen**
Inventions And Ideas . . . . . . . . . . . . . . . . . . . . . . . . . . . . 195

**Chapter Nineteen**
Injury Prevention Measures . . . . . . . . . . . . . . . . . . . . . . . 201

**Chapter Twenty**
When Left Is Right. . . . . . . . . . . . . . . . . . . . . . . . . . . . . . . . 219

**Frequently Asked Questions** . . . . . . . . . . . . . . . . . . . . . . 231

**Bibliography**. . . . . . . . . . . . . . . . . . . . . . . . . . . . . . . . . . . 239

# ACKNOWLEDGEMENTS

Books cannot be written and published without help. Where help comes can be found within families, co-workers, and friends (i.e. people you see every day). Then there are those found from phone calls, emails or regular mail that listened many evenings on the progress or lack of progress and always offered encouragement and questions leading to more answers found within this book. Many of my former co-workers also remain my friends through the WWW who continue to listen to my ideas which are frequently "out of the box." Thanks to Joan Bauch, RN, CCM, Vicky Kirby RN, CCM, Chakita Mann, RN, CCM., Sylvia Basak, Adjuster, Debra Levy, Vice President of the Southeast and Lydia Oliver, Supervisor, Denise Gray, Supervisor were co workers who were by my side when the patent idea emerged.

And for others who gave me advice Jackie Shrout, CRC and Eve Farr, Financial Consultant, many thanks. For computer help R. J. Grafton, Jeff Danick and Russell Cameron, Dale Brown, Mathew Monroe, John Hipp, Jeffrey Brown, Jay Agnew, Sherry Kennedy, Heather Wallace, Eric Brown, and Charles Grafton, thank you so much for going beyond what I asked for. Art work graphic design by Rae Dejur was indeed a "work of art". For their comments on keyboard training: Kathy Bakon. David Huckabay, many more thanks for graphics and production ideas.

For her suggestions and comments about the exercises shown, kudos and complements go to Dr. Delores Mangels and Gloria Payne. Exercise to prevent computer related injuries were also demonstrated by Dr. Abe Cardwell which will help many users with neck problems. A big thank you goes to CME Resources and Independent Computer Consultants Association (ICCA) who recognize the importance of this book. To Dr. John Robinton with One Call Medical for his review and comment, thanks also. For Sue Lutz whose belief in the importance of my messages to computer users, gave impetus to this project: so thanks for your efforts. Also to OSHA and BLS workers, and especially, Brett Besser, who always steered me in the right directions, thanks to all. Mrs. Blau and the Cortex publication deserve much of the credit by authorizing certain passages and tables to explain their research. Finally, CME Resources for publishing my CEU program "CARPAL TUNNEL SYNDROME" for healthcare professionals, I will be forever grateful.

# PART ONE

## COMPUTER WORKSTATION: WE HAVE A PROBLEM

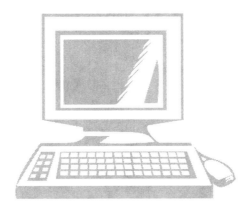

# INTRODUCTION

*When one door closes another one opens; but we so often look so long and so regretfully upon the closed door, that we do not see the ones which open for us.*

**Alexander Graham Bell**

## ALL COMPUTER USERS

Have you ever started a class with a bit of fear; not knowing what knowledge might bring? That fear appeared in my life the first hour while sitting in a computer class in 1998 in Las Vegas, Nevada. The class was the Internet for the Health Professional. Prior to the start of class, my education on computers and keyboards consisted of basic typing and word processing on my Apple 2E with one class of computer programming. Typing was not a problem but programming did not fit my learning mode. I wanted to learn how to use the Internet. Fear vanished after the first hour to be replaced by amazement as I gained access to the World Wide Web.

## THE INTERNET AND THE
## HEALTH CARE PROFESSIONAL

My future path appeared miraculously before my eyes. Clearly I saw a way to use my knowledge of research and writing, as communication techniques and strategies do fit my learning mode. The mechanics in searching the web and evaluating types of resources found were a perfect fit in my professional life. My health educator background and the types of books I write are all geared to help people with understanding learning. For example, my first book in 1978 was written for parents to help understand the differences between learning problems and learning disabilities. My second book was the development of the SOROL System (Starting Off: Right or Left). This system explained to start the process of learning to play tennis, you would need to know your dominance before you ever picked up a tennis racket as there was more to it than what hand do you write with or throw a ball with. This system was selected to be presented at the 1980 United States Professional Tennis Association Annual Convention in Las Vegas, Nevada. My fascination with the powers of the mind and how to outsmart the left brain with use of the hands continue to this day. Over the past eight years, I have worked all day, every day on my computer like so many working on medical case management claims. My mind is flooded with pop ups, ideas for helping my patients, my friends and family. Writing this book will help many people I do not know or will ever know. But there is self-fulfillment associated with these large scale plans put to paper. I copyrighted some of those ideas in 2002 along with a patent application in my spare time on my home computer. The culmination of those ideas was the development of training modules in power point for group presentations.

From working with spinal cord injury patients, I knew how quadriplegics were able to make use of computers with use of their eye blinks or breathe puffs to move the cursor in the early 90s. If you were having computer related work injuries, it seemed logical to use voice recognition should you be unable to use both hands. Then, if you were unable to use the right hand from overuse, then let us then use the left hand. That sounds simple. I knew direction-ality between the hands would be an issue. I did not know there would be not only a difference between the hands, but also a differ-ence between the fingers. So, this is how the story unfolds.

We all have dominance whether it is brain, hands, side, ears, eyes or feet. Now, how to use your dominance for productivity and longevity with computer keyboarding is the main focus of this book along with the exercises and education to overcome interference with the use of your genetic dominance and the selection of appropriate equipment such as input or wireless devices, voice recognition software and foot pedal options. This is assistive technology at a higher level with step by step tutorials leading to increased dexterity with the hands and fingers.

Microsoft uses Dexterity Training in their Business Solutions Visual C++ applications designs. Kung Fu trainers teach dexterity of the feet. This cross training acknowledges the requirements of both physical and mental conditioning. The website nimblefingers. com teaches typing games to improve dexterity. Other websites offer CAD and fighter pilot hand and finger dexterity. Not to be left out are websites that explain how a surgeon may improve dexterity with the use of virtual reality simulation in endoscopic and laser equipment. Also many websites offer soft rubber ball training for strengthening the hands.

Now in private practice in northwest Florida, I am writing down more of my ideas for computer users to improve their productivity at work, and then distribute the load of right hand computer usage to the left hand. Using my knowledge, skill and abilities, I have researched the web at length and our local universities libraries and found a need. That need is to develop a more sophisticated and educational system of keyboard set ups for not only the disabled population from their worker's compensation injuries but for the entire continuum of keyboard users, nationally and internationally. The plan has short term and long term capabilities to help solve the issue of computer related injuries.

What you will find as you read this book is information what researchers have to say about over use injuries due to use of computers. Research about the computer industry, the litigation against the industry, research about brain organization, and then how to train your non-dominant hand (the left) for use of a numerical data input or mouse device is the most important part of this book. Also you will find in the chapters are, how to select the appropriate devices based on your dominance and for those that you wish to help right along with you, this education and training.

Following training of the non preferred left hand, you will be able to alternate numerical data entry, assisting with lessening of repetitive data entry with your preferred right hand. Also mouse training is included. You may find the exercises shown to be more helpful than you could imagine, as you focus on what is in it for you.

## ERGONOMIC STRATEGIES

Just once in your life you may find that left is right and at the right time. This book is not meant to be an expose of the industry but an informative explanation of how you and for those you work with, may reduce your exposure to the overuse of your right hand through use of the computer or office machine or even your work station set up. You will learn techniques for your convenience or to increase productivity while at the same time, saving your hands, saving your money and perhaps, even saving your job. Many companies require employees to maintain high production levels with computers and especially numerical keypads without regard to effects of over use of a body part, especially the right hand side of the computer with the mouse, note pad, numerical keypad and insert and delete keys all located on that side. The arrangement described is over 2/3rds of the regular keyboard.

Look at your computer work station and you will see the same thing I see. And where is your telephone? Is it to your right? Hopefully it is on the left side, or better yet, have you thought about ear phone headsets? What about your writing hand? Are you a right handed or left handed writer with a pencil? If you work a great amount of time with a keypad or calculator and you are right handed consider purchasing a keypad or calculators that will fit your dominance, on the left side that is, while using your right hand for your usual writing. How do you accomplish the task or skill of using your left hand? The following pages will explain. You will be able to not only save money with knowing what computer devices to buy by eliminating trial and error purchasing but saving your hands from needless tapping on your computer keypads, just by reading this book carefully. The Bureau of Labor, prior to 2000, indicated 50% of computer users would have the dreaded Carpal Tunnel Syndrome. Microsoft acknowledges in their Resource Guide for Individuals with Dexterity Difficulties and Impairments using a standard keyboard or mouse among adult computer users in the USA, noting 1 in 4 (26%) will have problems that can be caused by a wide range of common illnesses and common accidents.

As you read through the chapters, you will find many answers to those questions. Probably many thoughts will come to you while learning to use your computer, so those thoughts will unfold for you, opening your eyes and finding solutions for your work station and also for those that you supervise or are responsible for. Yes, you can improve your productivity with training the left hand. What I am offering you, by reading this book, you will find a way to relieve your repetitive strain injury (RSI) or Carpal Tunnel Syndrome (CTS) by providing you a method to develop your non-dominant hand, suggestions about computer device equipment that will help as you learn how to revise your work station and accomplish the tasks you are paid to do. If you are not having any hand or finger complaints, I will show you how to help prevent these types of problems as you continue to use the PC computer.

Ergonomic injuries are attracting more attention for two reasons: they're becoming more numerous, and the cost — in worker compensation, medical bills, and lost productivity — is rising. Computer use is one of the numerous reasons for the increase in musculoskeletal disorders or repetitive stress injuries (RSI), such as Carpal Tunnel Syndrome. Finding answers through innovation and research is more than a past-time for me. Twenty years ago Quality Circles was a big item for teachers. For the past ten years empowering others has been a by-word to improve quality and safety. Three years ago, the term evidence-based came into fruition and this method teaches you to formulate and research questions as you progress. I have combined these two methods in solving the puzzle of computer related injuries. By reading this book, you will be able to answer questions for yourself and then help your colleagues at the office.

In the January 2004 edition of the NW Florida Daily News, I reviewed an advertisement seeking workers for a local bank listing an essential job requirement; "To be considered candidates, should have the ability to operate a 10-key calculator by touch, using the right hand." What about the left hander who must use the right handed computer keyboard/keypad? Is this discrimination? Do you need to be right handed to obtain a job in banking? Or does the left handed worker need to become a right hander with office equipment? This will be elaborated on in the last part of the book. The more scientific ergonomic strategies since 2000 are to 1) fit the job to the person not 2) make the person fit the job. Ask yourself this question? Is the company I work for number one or number two?

## AGGRAVATION AND WORK INJURIES IN COMPUTER LITIGATION

Over-use injuries are particularly noticeable among women shift workers who engage in data entry. Do the computer makers have negligent product liability for an improper overloaded design with the numerical keyboard on the right? This may well be the same for the companies that utilize the computer and regular keyboard and keypad with negligent failure to warn their employees of repetitive strain (RSI) and carpal tunnel syndrome (CTS).

In 1996, a Brooklyn court found DEC liable for $6 million for failure to place warning stickers on the computer. According to LexisNexis 5/17/04, "More than 25,600 CTS surgeries were performed in a single year." This is caused from "aggravation from repetitive movements, such as typing on a keyboard." From CTD News, more than 3000 RSI law suits are pending against keyboard manufacturers. Definitely, training programs are needed for high risk jobs.

From the website of dillinghammurphy.com, Mass Torts on the Immediate Horizon, due to repetitive stress syndrome cases, particularly carpal tunnel injuries and continuous subclinical trauma to the cervical spine, appear rampant at the workers' compensation level. Cases are defended vigorously but they will probably opt for some form of mass disposition. It is difficult to predict the future of this potential mass tort litigation according to the website. IBM, Apple and other PC manufacturers are the targets of a well-funded plaintiffs' bar from this article about litigation.

## RIGHTS OF INJURED WORKERS

Why is this meaningful to you? If you work in a large office with many workers involved at the computer workstation, not taking rest breaks throughout the day, working overtime and many of your coworkers having hand, finger, upper extremity pain or numbness, you may wish to discuss with your Human Resource Officer what can be done? Employers and their workers' compensation insurance companies have an obligation to inform Carpal Tunnel Syndrome sufferers of their right to benefits for work related injuries according to the chicagolegalnet.com web site.

Claims Adjusters at these insurance companies often do not have the expertise and will just deny the claim. The most painful part of Carpal Tunnel Syndrome is the pain usually is more severe at night and these individuals are not aware this condition is often related to their employment. Do not just walk away from this. If you do not get the right answer from your insurance company or your Human Resource Officer to help resolve the issue, you may wish to contact an attorney skilled in workers' compensation or product design flaws or your state workers compensation attorney general office for relief. There is a Workplace Injury Litigation Group at 303-830-0112 which may help you with your questions. Insurance companies have their own attorneys too and their sole responsibility is to protect the financial interests of the insurance group. Presently, 25% of all computer operators have Carpal Tunnel Syndrome and "estimates that by the year 2000, 50% of the entire workforce may be affected" was found in the statistics and disabling workers in epidemic proportions. Here it is 2009 and how many more of our and the world's computer workforce have developed this problem?

Alternative keyboards and peripherals solutions are being developed. This book will explain differences in human functional factors for computer keyboard and numerical pad users. These user set ups for right handed and left handed users of computers with numerical keyboards must be different due to the individual brain organization of computer users. Some keyboard users have developed muscle and tendon diseases due to a medical condition, some to work related overuse or repetition and some, some of both.

Frequently this places the computer user out of work whether work related or the recreational at home computer user. The search for the keyboard to success has already begun. By reviewing new and old computer patents, the internet, searches for new electronic equipment, including programmable keyboards and keypads plus wireless keyboards and keypads and hundreds of books on how to deal with computer related Carpal Tunnel Syndrome or Repetitive Strain Injury, it is difficult to even keep up with changes in the industry. Only employers can change occupational environments to decrease its incidence of these problems. But, computer IT companies will be the developers of new designs but the methods by Health Educators and Trainers (like me).

## EARLY DEVELOPMENT OF THE COMPUTER

The abacus was first used in 500 B.C. to use as a basic arithmetic. While working in Tokyo, Japan, I was amazed at how fast people and students could use this method of calculation. In the 20s, the mechanical calculator, the slide rule was introduced. Fewer than ten computers existed in the 1940s. From the Computer Continuum book by Laukner and Linter, these authors ask "how have we allowed an inanimate machine to become so influential?" Computers help us perform repetitive tasks, calculate, manipulate numbers, store and receive information. Now we have scales and calculators, wireless communication and network access.

The development of the computer goes back to 1936 with Konrad Zuse who invented the first freely programmable computer. During the interim improvements were made, then in 1953 IBM entered into history with the 701 EDPM. Along came the chip in 1958 developed by Jack Kilby and Robert Noyce. Then, the mouse and Windows followed in 1964. You may have wondered how the mouse got its name. Supposedly, the mouse was named, as the tail came out of the end. The Internet was a decided jump in 1969 leading to the floppy disk by Alan Shugart and IBM. The IBM PC home computer was on the market in 1981. Apple Macintosh came in with your computer in 1984, not to be outdone by IBM and others. Microsoft Windows made an impact in 1985 leading to worldwide development of these products and devices.

One of the web news sources I use is the ergoweb.com. This is "The Trusted Source for Ergonomics News." Their December 13, 2004 edition asks "How Does a Keyboard Affect Comfort and Productivity?" The article discusses computer workers and "that any amount of time spent with a keyboard could end up with the same result: workers who report some degree of hand/wrist or elbow discomfort. So what can a workplace do to make computer tasks more comfortable for workers? Invest in keyboards and peripherals which can help improve both short-term and long-term comfort as well as productivity."

In testimony before the Senate about the PC technology industry on 2/12/04, Alan Greenspan stated: We are at 10% capacity as business does not know what to do with their technology and it takes 6 months to 2 years to outline a course of action. Given today underscores the need for aggressive action in the area of technology. We must all become an active part of the solution. By identifying the problem of over use injures with computer and numerical keypad users, not to assign blame but more importantly how we can improve the process of productivity in business. To preserve our system we must correct the problem and the solution begins with each one of us.

## ERGONOMICS AND FACTS WITH SUPPORT WEB SITES

In my opinion, our continued dependency on computers demand that companies become appropriately educated in injury prevention and provide ergonomically correct and safer computer working conditions. Research states "those 100,000 to 300,000 new carpal tunnel/computer injuries per year." And what about the current issue of outsourcing of computer jobs internationally? Are we passing the buck of our computer problems to other nations? From recent news stories internationally, some US companies have sold their computers with monitors and keyboards to Asian countries and will rely on software and peripheral sales. Asian countries, from my sources, do not have the tough Workers' Compensation or patent laws which American workers and companies enjoy.

Is this important? Absolutely. For the past few years OSHA lists Carpal Tunnel Syndrome and other over use injuries as the costliest disease or process nationwide. The outcome of these findings will have far reaching effects internationally.

New systems of operations will be developed, I feel, as a result of class action law suits against businesses, corporations, computer and office machine companies.

What I believe is the answer, for older systems, is a numerical key pad input device placed on the left side of the keyboard. This would essentially become a dual system of keypads. How the dual system numbers location setup is based on the person's dominance. In July of 2002, I copyrighted some of my ideas to reduce occupational injuries for workers but for the future, we need to include the dual numerical keypad for use in schools and universities. We need to educate all computer users to avoid this problem. For those of us in health occupations, this is cost containment. Also I recommend to my patients and readers of this book TIFAQ.com and the Fentek Industries website to read what is available in ergonomics and facts pertaining, to help understand what had happened to them and they were not alone with this problem. You will find mental support for yourself and others just by reading this book.

Fentek makes a left-handers keyboard but that is not the entire answer. How do you know what keypad numbers location to choose? Should the numbers go left to right, or right to left? Do you need to buy both and then try and figure out what is best for you? Now, a Multimedia Number Pad has been developed but that is not the answer either.

None of these keyboards explain why you would wish to buy one or the other. This is trial and error purchasing which does not fit the ergonomics solutions of today for professionals. Companies are making ergonomic changes in the mouse, keyboard design and devices but not until now has a long term solution been proposed or invented. A utility patent application was filed and issued 8/14/2007 and is the basis for the training method found in this book.

Smart businesses are not waiting for regulation or lawsuits to prompt action geared to preventing such repetitive motion injuries, i.e. Carpal Tunnel Syndrome (CTS).

According to records from Brooklyn, NY, 1996, a court awarded three women with Carpal Tunnel Syndrome 6 million dollars for a failure to warn sticker not placed on the computer. If you have a newer keyboard, check with your safety guide enclosed or some statement. Is there a warning through use of the product?

The technology company that acquires the rights to license my patent and training method will have a new way of looking at your computer work station. What I envision in the future, as you open your new computer, there will be a CD included for your dual keyboard/keypad. The number locations will already be downloaded with a switch to determine which number direction for your keypad. Or, the mouse training too if you decide to change the mouse to the left hand side of your computer or even have a dual system set up. This is not a far-fetched idea because Apple introduced their new 2.0 system for iPods in 2008 using gestures of the hands and/or fingers for your use in their operating system.

## SCOPE OF THE PROBLEM

According to the Occupational Safety and Health Administration (OSHA) 1.8 million workers are affected by a musculoskeletal disorder (MSD) each year. In 2000, the federal agency recently concluded public hearings on a proposed rule that would mandate that nearly every U.S. Company implement a formal ergonomic program focused on musculoskeletal disorders documented in the workplace.

And according to the American Medical Association, work-related injuries are a major cause of disability and death in the United States. High injury risk jobs include ones that expose you to chemicals, radiation, vibration, dusts, and loud noise. However, office workers experience work-related injuries too. Carpal Tunnel Syndrome is most common in people who have jobs that have repetitive hand motion and involve vibratory tools, like typewriters or computers. This injury causes a tingling/numbness in the thumb, index, and sometimes middle finger. People who sit at a desk or work on a computer all day are more likely to have back problems and headaches.

I trust you will pay close attention to the exercises, training and education to overcome dominance interference and the selection of appropriate equipment and devices for your work station. The solution for this dilemma of work place injuries through overuse of computers is to review the chapters so you will understand dominance factors, then to learn how to use the non dominant hand with the ideas expressed during the training and education portion. My style of learning is systematic, taking tasks or parts in order. But, if you are not systematic, whole learning instead of in parts, well, jump right in, just do it. Put your book on the left side, propped up with your document holder, open up the chapters on training and education and go from there. After training, you will need to go back to pick up the rest of the parts to answer your questions. But for those of us, part to part learner, sit back and enjoy the ride through why you need to make some changes (redesign) at your workstation.

First we will explain the important points about Carpal Tunnel Syndrome and Repetitive Strain Injuries, and then we will travel with the Table of Contents as your road map through information covering working postures, seating, document holders, mouse and other pointing devices, telephones, keyboard and input devices, monitors, work area, accessories and general ideas. Few computer users do not know or understand the power that is found in their hands. This book will explain those facts. I have formatted the rest of the chapters with websites which will help you as you educate yourself and how to formalize your plan for a safer computer workstation.

## THE SEVEN STEPS TO KEYBOARDING FOR SUCCESS ARE TO CLIMB THE EDUCATION LADDER

- Know the alternative solutions to reduce computer-related injuries
- Understand the risks in your job or occupation
- Complete the two workstation checklists from OSHA
- Review the exercises and warm-up and rest break regimens

- Identify your dominance for the Dual Numerical Keyboard
- Start Dexterity Training with use of the numerical keypad and the mouse for left hand usage
- Read the office safety training suggestions

# CHAPTER ONE

*The most likely way for the world to be destroyed, most experts agree, is by accident. That's where we come in; we're computer professionals. We cause accidents.*

**Nathan Borenstein**

## CARPAL TUNNEL SYNDROME AND OTHER MUSCLE AND TENDON DISORDERS

If you are an injured worker or a safety officer requesting a needs assessment for any assistive technology device or assistance with computers please visit the website www.tricare.mili/cap/wsm. There are so many people with a disability; the federal government offers initiatives to hire for positions, even if you are a student. Microsoft, IBM and Apple are familiar names for computer users and support many organizations. The Assistive Technology Industry Association or ATIA is one of the larger groups that educate device designers for hardware and software featuring innovative products or training programs for people with disabilities including people with Carpal Tunnel Syndrome. Workplace Musculoskeletal Disorders (WMSD) account for 34% of all lost workday injuries or illnesses.

How serious is the Carpal Tunnel Problem is best answered by this from our own Bureau of Labor. Currently, Carpal Tunnel Syndrome (CTS) affects over 8 million Americans in the work force and it is "the chief occupational hazard of the 90"s." In 1992, the Bureau of Labor Statistics found that while women account for 45% of all workers, they experienced nearly 2/3's of all work—

related CTS and RSI. There are numerous terms used to describe these types of disorders. You will see RSI, MSD, CTS used frequently. During this chapter, you will begin to understand how the terms are used how the diagnosis is made from the symptoms of these disabling conditions.

The intended readers of this book are people who use the computer every day in the course of their work whether you work in an office, home office or on the road with your lap top. You may be a corporate nurse, case manager (field or telephonic), vocational evaluator, disability specialist, vocational counselor, physician, psychologist, accountant, bank worker, writer, financial consultant, Design Engineer in space exploration, CAD Operator, Architect, real estate personnel or anyone that uses a keypad, calculator or mouse. Let us not leave out human resource and safety officers who definitely need this information found in these pages.

From the Medical Library website of the American Medical Association, medem.com "The Carpal Tunnel is the area under a ligament in front of the wrist." If you will open your left hand and with your right hand with your index finger, trace an area from the outside of your palm to the inside of the palm and into the thumb. This is the ligament that covers the carpal tunnel. With the same hand but with the four fingers (not the thumb) start at the thumb, 1st, 2nd, 3rd and 4th fingers coming down toward the inside of the wrist and that will be the tunnel that holds the tendons, tendon sheaths and median nerve which are inside the tunnel. "Repetitive movements of the hand and wrist can cause inflammation of structures." "The inflammation may compress this nerve, producing numbness, tingling, and pain in the first three fingers and the thumb side of the hand-a condition known as Carpal Tunnel Syndrome."

If you need a laminated listing and pictures of the spinal cord, hands, finger and tendons, you can write or request to mdmonline. com or go to diatri.net.

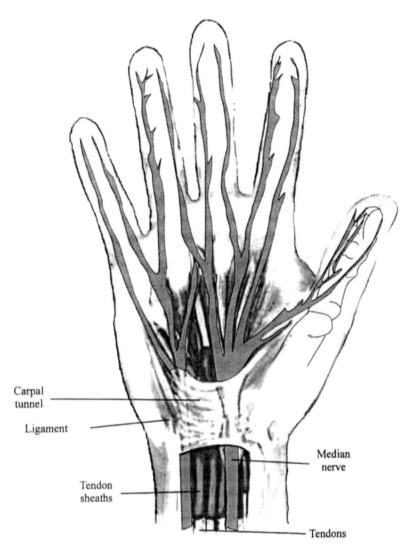

*Carpal Tunnel Anatomy*

In a seminar in Las Vegas, Nevada in 1999 by Dr. Michael Erdil (Health Direct, Inc.), alluded that "the past decade has seen a marked rise in reported cases of upper extremity cumulative trauma disorders." He mentions muscular and tendon "strain and most notably, Carpal Tunnel Syndrome" to be a major disorder. OSHA "estimates that work-related musculoskeletal disorders in the US account for over 600,000 injuries and illnesses that are serious enough to result in days away from work (34 percent of all lost workday injuries report the BLS)." "It is estimated that employers spend as much as $15–18 billion a year on direct costs" for these types of injuries from the web site osha.gov.

## TERMS

In a seminar in Atlanta, 2002, Dr. Arthur Simon, Hand Specialist, discussed these conditions "referring to a category of physical signs and symptoms due to repeated, long term musculoskeletal injuries where the causes appear to be related to repetitive work." The CTD's "are a result of years of small microtrauma (tears in the muscle or tendon)." Dr. Simon listed these terms for better understanding.

**RSI** — repetitive strain injury

**CTS** — Carpal Tunnel Syndrome — a common problem in office practice and is increasingly recognized in many occupations. This condition is compression and entrapment of the median nerve found in the hand.

**CTD** — cumulative trauma disorder-characterized by forceful, repetitive hand tasks

**Tendonitis** — a form of tendon inflammation (swelling) that happens when a muscle/tendon unit is repeatedly tensed

**DeQuervain's** — the tendon becomes constricted in the over lying tendon sheath

**Trigger finger** — occurs when the tendon sheath of the index finger is swollen so that the tendon becomes locked in the sheath

**Tennis elbow (lateral epicondylitis)** — tendonitis that occurs on the outside of the elbow

We talk about the fingers and the wrist, what about the thumb? Due to the rising use of laptop computers, both thumbs are frequently used to use the cursor and enter spaces (touch pads). I have had several claimants with both trigger finger (index finger) and DeQuervain's disease (the thumb) which required lengthy treatment.

There are three basic categories of RSI according to diatri.net with the name given to a group of conditions that are caused when too much stress is placed on a joint. Most RSI's occur in the upper extremities. RSI's involving nerves, those involving tendons, muscles and soft tissues and those involving the vascular or blood vessel system are listings from this radiology company.

The Neurology Channel on the web indicates the primary risk factor is a history of another musculoskeletal disorder. When you use your wrist repetitively such as an accountant, writer, computer operator or programmer, this condition develops. Even if you have a medical disease and your computer work has aggravated the condition, it does not mean your pain is not work related.

What are the conservative methods for treating CTS and RSI? The standard methods to date are wrist splints, hot and cold compresses, exercise and physical therapy. Aspirin and/or corticosteroids are the usual medications. Your doctor will ask you about your symptoms, review your history, do his physical exam using Phalen's maneuver and Tinel's sign and may request nerve conduction testing, EMG, MRI or Sonography.

Two of the researchers in computer related injuries are Pascarelli E.F. and Hsu. (2002) who studied "four hundred eighty five patients whose chief complaints were work related pain and other symptoms. They received a comprehensive upper-body clinical evaluation to determine the extent of their illness. The group had a mean age of 38.5 years. Sixty-three percent of patients were females. Seventy percent were computer users, 28% were musicians and 2% were others engaged in repetitive work." "A majority sought care within 30 months with the greatest number of them seeking care before 12 months. Fifty nine percent of subjects were still working when seen despite increasing pain and symptoms such as weakness, numbness, tingling, and stiffness" (1–21).

You can see from the symptom list, you could have several problems rolled into one from overuse of the computer. The "number of patients with positive clinical findings in this study lends weight to the concept that posture related neurogenic symptoms are a key factor in the cascading series of physical events that characterize this illness." These researchers concluded "a comprehensive upper-body examination produces findings that cannot be obtained through laboratory tests and surveys alone and lays the ground work for generating hypotheses about the etiology of work related upper-extremity disorders that can be tested in controlled investigations." This particular group of researchers and physicians are Orthopedic, Physical Medicine and Internal Medicine specialists at Columbia University in New York. From reading Dr. Pascarelli's book about RSI, written in 1994, I could tell his patients were primarily computer related or musician related hand injuries. Later in this book, you will see the importance of these comparisons.

"When exactly can Carpal Tunnel Syndrome be considered work related" is the topic of Falkiner S., Myers and Anz (2002) at New South Wales, Australia. These researchers write of the primary risk factors in the development of CTS are: being a woman of menopausal age, obesity or lack of fitness, diabetes or having a family history of diabetes, osteoarthritis of the carpometacarpal joint of the thumb, smoking, and lifetime alcohol intake. Pregnancy is also considered as a risk factor. Causation of CTS in most cases, these authors believe work acts as the "last straw." You may ask, why obesity? Anything (extra fat) that increases pressure in the carpal tunnel may contribute to CTS.

If you believe you may have CTS or RSI and see your physician and ask for a laboratory test to confirm, your physician may not agree to this. According to van Dijk M. Reitsma, Fischer and Sanden (2003), "at present, there is insufficient evidence for routine laboratory screening for concurrent conditions in all newly diagnosed CTS patients." This study concluded the "prevalence of diabetes mellitus, hypothyroidism, and rheumatoid arthritis are higher in CTS patients."

All of the adjusters that I worked with knew of my interest in following computer related injuries and with the approval with the V. P. of our regional office, gave my recommendations to reduce computer related problems which included education with the use of several websites. Before a claim was referred to me, the Adjuster generally talked to the Employer and frequently their Safety Officer. Following a particular claim whereby the worker was unable to use the right hand at work at her keyboard per doctor's order, I knew there was more that could be done for these types of worker injuries at the work station. I set out to find out this could be done with this claim, training the left hand for keying data using the keypad or the calculator.

In an email response to my questions to Dr. John Robinton, Physiatrist with One Call Medical, Dr. Robinton reviewed some of my research and stated my "approach to the issues identified with computer overuse are a reasonable approach to this problem." Dr. Robinton is known for his work with muscle testing using EMG and NCS associated with these types of injuries.

Results from Medline indicate that litigation does affect patient utilization of health care and increase the workload of the Physician. This increases the cost of healthcare too. Is your case in litigation? If so, here are more solutions to RSI and CTS. You may wish to share this book's information with your attorney. There are more web sites that have workplace solutions for repetitive stress injuries.

Log on to www.ctdnews.com. Some of their advice points to how overtime can increase your risk and how return to work rehab in a real work environment can be more effective than off site. If you are a supervisor and wish to help your workers, discuss this book with your personnel office staff. You may have just found the right ergonomics solution for your department.

## STATISTICS

A news bulletin from the United States Department of Labor regarding Computer and Internet Use at Work in 2001 stated 72.3 million persons used a computer at work. Highlights from that bulletin included the proportion of workers who used a computer varied greatly by occupation. Also more women than men use the computer. In private-sector industries, workers in finance, insurance, and the real estate industry had the highest rates of computer use at 81.4 percent. The most important statistic from this bulletin was of the 72.3 million computer users, 62.3 percent worked with spreadsheets or databases. Secondly, in terms of occupations, workers in managerial and professional specialty occupations 70.3 percent use spreadsheets or databases. For the complete report, go to the website of www.bls.gov/news.release. The average Federal government cost (medical & Worker's Compensation costs) for a carpal tunnel syndrome case is $8,799.00.

According to the Southern California Orthopedic Institute, CTS occurs more often in women than men, by a ratio of 3 to 1 and usually between the ages of 30 to 50 years doing forceful types of work of a repetitive nature such as typists, accountants and writers. They suggest appropriate modification in activities as the first line of defense. "Computer occupations for all workers are projected to have some of the steepest gains between 2000 and 2010." This article enforces that women need to recognize that in addition to paying well in the computer industry, projections for further growth indicate software and applications for information technology continue to have a substantial impact on employment opportunities in the United States.

Girls and women need in-depth knowledge of the theories and principles of science and mathematics acquired while in school or university. Should women continue to become computer scientists and systems analysts through completion of a bachelor's degree or higher, their increase for these jobs will make up more than three out of ten of these jobs. Among natural scientists, women represented 51.6 percent of medical scientists.

So you see it is important to prepare for the future in the management of data with use of both hands for numerical data entry. Up to now employment of women has lagged in most of the high tech jobs that show promise for future growth. The challenges for women are to find more pathways into the occupations that will show promise by exploring educational and training opportunities that will lead to high-tech careers.

Johnny Evans, a writer for TechWorld (5/6/08) states work-related RSI cases are at an all time high and the cost to business continue to spiral upwards of 30 percent in the last year. Microsoft claims the rapidly emerging trend of mobile-working i.e., office-based employees working on the move for over an hour per day than they did two years ago are the driving factor behind this alarming upward climb. The costs to businesses are US $600 million in lost working hours. Research suggests one of the main factors behind the increasing numbers were companies not being aware of the high risk of RSI with 68 percent did nothing when employees reported problems. Microsoft advises that companies do not replace existing office equipment with more ergonomic hardware that can reduce these types of worker injuries.

There are so many new products on the market you can become an expert by paying close attention to the solutions already mentioned in the first part of this book. The last part of the book is devoted to prevention of computer related CTS. So, what I am asking you to do now is to assess your work station, wrist positions and repetitive hand movements, modify your layout, and altering the existing method for doing some of your job tasks. These work-sheets/checklists can be found at the OSHA website under eTool or the Ergo Guide at the TRICARE website and I suggest you pull up those free documents, and print them out and complete them.

So many books, studies, web sites have written of these types of injuries and what the medical community and pharmaceutical answers for the pain and inflammation have developed- that I am trying to stay away from what has already been done. The best person to give medical advice, diagnoses and treatment is your doc-tor or other qualified medical professional. Please do not try and diagnose yourself as you finish reading all the chapters in this book. If you are having problems, you will know exactly how to go about seeking advice from your employer before seeing an occupational specialist or your medical provider.

You should know now what to look for in job risks, some of the alternative solutions to hand and wrist injuries and through com-pletion of the workstation checklists, the way to begin making the changes that will help you gain productivity and with that, longev-ity from computer usage.

# CHAPTER TWO

*To err is human — and to blame it on a computer is even more so.*

**Robert Orben**

## TYPES OF TREATMENT

Ergonomic related injuries account for $20 billion in Worker's Compensation treatment costs each year. The importance of this information already provided to you should stand tall in your mind by now. There will always be controversy about these hand/arm/fingers/shoulder complaints, the cause and most importantly what to do about it. Just ask someone who has the tingling, burning, cramping pain in the middle of the night and they must resort to wearing wrist splints at night. Don't' forget to include the computer worker who is hard pressed to keep up assignments that must shake out her hands from the cramping and drawing up the hand and finger muscles and then resort to crying at their work station. Often a trial of different types of medications to relieve the pain is offered but you cannot take narcotics at work so anti-inflammatory medications are given.

Training programs always begin with all the items needed at the computer work station and all the dimensions used for correct postures for the body, the chair and all the items around you. Depending upon what your job requires and what you need could be two different things. You will hear more about risks associated with your job. Did you know that insurance rate is based on risk of injury?

McDiarmid M., Oliver, Ruser and Guser (2000) in their study of "male and female workers lost time from work due to CTS argued that men and women doing the same work tasks would have similar rate of CTS." They used BLS statistics in 6 high risk occupations. Variable job tasks exist within 5 of the 6 high risk occupational titles. The data entry keyers, which "require a single physical task, had a risk rate ratio of 1.06, more than double the other occupations." They also state that "women are over represented in jobs at high risk for CTS" (23–32). Cail F. and Aptel (2003) in their study of "biomechanical stresses between CAD and data entry workers found that complaints emerged from workers upper limbs were linked to input devices." They also found that "grip forces exerted when using the keyboard and mouse was higher in CAD than in data entry workers. (235–55)."

Dr. Pascarelli (1993) in his study of soft tissue injuries related to use of the computer keyboard believed that harmful inefficient keyboard styles (intrinsic ergonomic factors) and changes in the workstation (extrinsic ergonomic factors) must be addressed and corrected by a combination of factors including technique retraining and education. Beredjiklian P., Bozentka, Steinberg, and Bernstein (2000) evaluated the source and content of orthopaedic information on the Internet reviewing information available on Carpal Tunnel Syndrome. Their conclusion is that the information on the Internet is "of limited quality and poor informational value." They further concluded "the public and medical communities need to be aware of these limitations so that the quality of medical information on the World Wide Web can be improved." In other words, look carefully at the site if there are commercial products sold on the site and what academic organization is providing the information (1540–3).

Computers and health hazards will continue due to computer intensive work styles causing the nerve disorder of the wrist. The most frightening of the CTS statistics from BLS is up to 36% of all

Carpal Tunnel Syndrome patients require unlimited medical treatment and only 23% of all Carpal Tunnel Syndrome patients were able to return to their previous professions following surgery.

From the February 2005 issue of Arthritis and Rheumatism, in a trial conducted at several hospitals in Madrid, Spain, patients were injected with corticosteroids had more improvement in function and reported less pain after three months than those that had surgery. Look at all of your options before throwing up your hands to select your treatment. There are a few books on the market today on Carpal Tunnel Syndrome but not a complete and informative way to reduce your exposure from repetitive use of the keyboard and keypad. Some of these books and tapes will only give you exercises to do but not what this book has to offer you.

What I am offering you, is a way to stay at work, change your work station to fit your needs and to train your left hand for numerical data entry or move your mouse to the left side of your work station plus do preventative simple hand and wrist warm-ups at the start of the work day and rest break with upper body exercises.

Just as the notable breast cancer surgeon, Deborah Axelrod acknowledged the need to look beyond pills and traditional medical interventions to reduce the chance that disease will recur, we need to look more closely at our computer workstation and make the decision to use your genetic dominance in the use of the keyboard, calculator and mouse and not as the so-called "preference" as advocated in OSHA's eTool in 2004. Preferences are those that are found in the generic set up in the classroom or bought and sold in a box by computer makers and resellers. A better word, rather than preference, is either trait or genetic dominance. The purpose of this book is to explain why an alternative solution is needed for those computer users who have developed repetitive strain injuries and a different direction in work habits to overcome those injuries. Take responsibility for your workstation at the office or at home and help prevent work related computer injuries.

# PART TWO

---

## CLEAR AND
## CONVINCING EVIDENCE

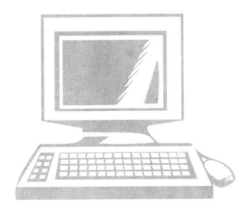

# CHAPTER THREE

*Information technology and business are becoming inextricably interwoven. I don't think anybody can talk meaningfully about one without the talking about the other.*

**Bill Gates**

## FACTORS TO CONSIDER

The computer is a vital tool in many different occupations. However, long periods of working at a computer can increase the chance of developing an injury according to the Computer Health website. Muscle and joint pain, overuse injuries of the upper limbs and eyestrain can result from inappropriate computer use. But, for your computer health, risks can be reduced or eliminated with proper work space design, improved posture and good working habits. Through repeated finger and hand movements, you are at risk for the development of work related injuries. How can this book help you? By explaining about your dominance, (whether you are right handed or left handed) , you will learn how to select a mouse, a keypad device and how to train your non preferred left hand to use the numerical keypad or calculator. Computer technicians with the giant corporations are grappling with alternative solutions to assist in solving the problems of work related computer use. These are the occupations from IT technology that have learned how to break into the tech industry by specializing in one of these fields: IT Manager, Software Engineer, Programmer, Web Developer, and Systems Analyst.

## CTS #1 REPORTED MEDICAL PROBLEM

Carpal Tunnel Syndrome is the #1 reported medical problem accounting for 50% of all work-related injuries according to the Dept. of Labor. As you read along, you will find out whether your job is high risk or low risk for the development of CTS. As a Nurse Case Manager for the past fifteen years and over eleven years of workers compensation medical management experience, I have been faced with helping injured workers within the framework of available ergonomic programs. But the diagnosis given to many computer users through the medical system of work related injuries are often perplexing.

## THE JOB AND THE COMPUTER APPEAR TO BE ONE

By working with family members, employers, attorneys, physicians or other professionals (Vocational Evaluators, Psychologists), we provide the necessary services with either face to face or telephonic communication, then writing and documenting all that is said and done with various computer software systems and programs. We obtain job descriptions, medical records, authorize medical treatment, and associated diagnostic testing. Also we develop medical strategies and give the provider information necessary to facilitate a return to work plan.

## COST CONTAINMENT EFFORTS AND
## WORKERS COMPENSATION

In some jurisdictions, Nurses are allowed to direct care and to challenge providers by suggesting cost effective treatment alternatives. This book identifies and suggests the possibility of a Work Hardening program to benefit the worker, the employer and the insurance company. Rather than go out on workers' compensation leave with 2/3rds of your pay when you must rest your right hand and arm, why not stay on the job and train your non preferred hand for some of your tasks? At the Hughston Clinic in Columbus, Ga., Dr. David

C. Rehak writes of the benefits of work hardening programs. These programs allow employees to return to work in part-time positions or in a modified-duty program. These programs halt the effects of atrophy and the psychological effects of depression that come from being out of work. Dr. Rehak recommends, "keep the daily routine by keeping in mind that rest is not always best."

## OCCUPATIONS LISTED AS COMPUTER USERS

What is your job now? Are you in a health occupation? Do you need to use pharmacological dosages, concentrations or body mass index calculation? Do you use an electronic calculator to interpret record results of various spreadsheet fundamentals? Do you use database management software and manipulate data or create new databases? Are you a Grade 8 Math Teacher having your students use calculators to explore patterns among fraction/decimal relationships? Do you work at a car rental return or a sheet metal worker in construction using a hand calculator? Did you find your job from those questions? If you need more specific information about your job or occupation, write to www.oshstaff

There are many occupations that require supervisory and management functions. These jobs often require accounting, marketing and personnel work. Tellers receive and pay out money. New Accounts Clerks working in banks interview persons wishing to open accounts and assist in preparing forms. Transit Clerks record and sort items for mailing to insure routing and collection. Loan Interviewers, Credit Authorizers, Credit Checkers all use calculators as a part of the job. Clerks in loan and credit departments prepare and distribute bank statements all requiring use of a calculator. Insurance adjusters, examiners and investigators calculate benefit payments. Right along with other personnel in insurance are Claims Clerks and Examining Clerks.

If you work at a state facility, you may be a Welfare Eligibility Worker or Interviewer, or Clerical Investigator. Or in a state court system as a Court Clerk or Municipal Clerk you may keep fiscal records and accounts? And then there are Statistical Clerks who probably perform actuarial computations using algebra and trigonometry graphs. Persons working in accounting offices are Bookkeepers, Accounting Clerks and Auditing Clerks. They must be accurate with their figures and calculations. Payroll functions require computing fees, charges, invoices calculating rates for many types of records. Other job titles in these organizations are Billing, Posting and Calculating Machine Operators. By operating bookkeeping machines they copy and post data completing records of transactions.

Computer Operators monitor and control electronic data. Peripheral EDP Operators need to tabulate other machines. Data entry keyers, whether composing or not composing, must use numeric data. Even if you are a Meter Reader for a utilities company, you will be recording data on a hand held calculator or portable laptop PC. Many occupations are entry level. You may be able to develop the necessary skills of data management through on the job training in records processing occupations according to the jobbank.usa.com. Payroll clerks, billing clerks and bookkeeping, accounting auditing clerks should have a strong aptitude for numbers. To move up in these types of jobs requires focus on productivity.

Most records processing clerks enter data into a computer system and perform basic analysis of the data. This could include medical record clerks, hotel and motel clerks and reservation and transportation ticket agents. If you are taking mathematics 9–12, you will use a graphing calculator according to Kathryn.Wright@k12.sd. us.

"Techretaries" take care of business according to the Freedom News Wire article by Kerry McGinley 5/22/05. It's been years since the title "secretary" went out of vogue. The increasing demand for administrative staff to keep abreast of changing technology and computer skills, 'techretary' may be a more appropriate moniker.

McGinley also writes many companies now are looking for the administrative staff to be the first to try out new technology tools and assist their teams in learning new technology tools.

Computer Assisted Design or CAD software is used by 25 million people all over the world according to Graeme Philipson in the SMH bulletin 3/4/05. These are just some of the jobs requiring the use of the numeric keypad or a numerical calculator. I cannot stress enough; this is not just a United States of America dilemma but an international one.

## RSI STATISTICS

Presently, 25% of all computer operators have Carpal Tunnel Syndrome and estimates that by the year 2000, 50% of the entire workforce may be affected. This is from the Bureau of Labor Statistics written at that time. Now, from the statistics known of over 73 million computer users when I started this book and six months later, a radio broadcast with news that 53 million new PC's were sold in the USA in 2004 makes me realize the importance of the information I am sharing with you. From 1975 through 2005, 400 million computers have been sold. In 2006, 60 million new computers were made and already in November 2007 over 60 million more have been made. A better statistic is in the past year over 18 million computers have been manufactured. Isn't it time you became an expert in how to save your hands and begin to think about your longevity and productivity at your work station?

# CHAPTER FOUR

*Man is still the most extraordinary computer of all.*

John F. Kennedy

## ALTERNATIVE SOLUTIONS

Since the majority of the populations worldwide are right handed, the right hand is generally used for the regular numerical keyboard on computers or business machines. Often during treatment for CTS or RSI by their physician, work limitations will be given, i.e. no use of right arm or right hand and wrist. These computer users are often out of work as their employers cannot provide another system or adaptation of the numerical keyboard as a part of their work limitations.

Many companies have production guidelines which must be met. Companies like banks, financial institutions, credit card companies, health care and insurance companies are large users of the computer and keypad. Many of these companies have two to three shifts of workers to accomplish production levels within their guidelines. As a result of these actions, there may be negligent liability from the design of the computer and keyboard but also liability with failure to warn on the part of the employers with large numbers of employees with these types of complaints, lost time, lost wages and some lost jobs by using the overloaded right side of keyboard. The average annual cost to an employer for altering a workstation is $150.00.

The computer electronics industry is rapidly developing changes for keyboard users but they do not tell you why.

Much of the push is from our own Government who follow workplace injuries. For every injury at work, the injury is logged for OSHA to review. If there are too many, then the company is contacted and safety measures followed to reduce those types of injuries. When OSHA finds violations in the workplace, they are categorized as serious, willful, repeat and other-than-serious. The hazards of your workplace are supposed to be posted on Employee Bulletin Boards. "Strong, fair, and effective enforcement, using mechanisms such as Site Specific Targeting (SST) and the Enhanced Enforcement Program (EEP), is a key component in achieving" the goal of decreasing workplace injuries. OSHA will focus in the future their activities with outreach, education and enforcement. When reviewing information at the web site of the United States Patent Office (USPO) regarding new applications for patents, you can easily understand the history of the computer and keyboard/keypad innovations with all of the improvements being made. Layouts of keys and functionality provided by those keys are ever changing.

Computer electronics companies are developing programs for people with disabilities. There are a variety of tools available for individuals with upper extremity amputations. On October 17, 2006, Public Law 109-364 was passed, allowing Service members injured while on active duty to retain all assistive technology and services provided from CAP upon separation from active duty. This has permitted many Service members to continue their education or return to the workforce with the use of the CAP-provided assistive technology. For more information about the CAP Wounded Service Member Initiative, please visit tricare.mil/cap/wsm.

In the final accounting by our USPO for 2005, there were 10,366 patents from the top five companies. IBM, Canon, Hewlett Packard, Matsushita Electric Industrial Co., Ltd, and Samsung Electronics head the list. Our Secretary of Commerce for Intellectual Property, Jon Dudas, has plans IN 2006 "to ensure that U. S. intellectual property protection remains the best in the world" because of our "tremendous ingenuity." In 2007 the patent office was recruiting students to think of patents as a way to sell their ideas.

There were numerous complaints written about the problems associated with the original 83 key layout with the cramped physical groupings. Since the QWERTY keyboard was introduced to improve the layout of the keys, this attempt accommodated the mirror-image symmetry of the hands or to conform to the spacing and agility of individual fingers. In my research, I could not find the answer of why, but this was a good try in recognizing differences in the use of two hands at the keyboard. Dvorak, a Design Engineer accomplished in Human Engineering in the 1940s, developed the Dvorak Keyboard which would favor the right hander thus taking away the advantage of the left handed typist. At first there were no dedicated cursor or navigation keys. Many computers users did not like the left side function keys. IBM continued to make changes and improvements with better physical groupings. When the enhanced 101 keyboard layout was introduced with the extra numeric keypad keys (enter and /), the design change helped many data entry workers.

The 104 Windows Keyboards have special purpose key designs: new audio and mouse controls and Internet shortcuts. Now, programmable keyboards and devices allow the user to define individual keys; so again progress is being made. But not enough progress has been made. Innovators in computer design are looking beyond hands and fingers, moving up to the arms. A new adaptation of the keyboard works around the lower forearm and requires use of the biceps muscle in the upper arm from the website at tiger. com.

As computer design inventors improve the networking within the computer and the computer user with their energy fields, a whole new world will open up for computer makers. The experimental computer has been devised to father a long line of biological computers to create computers that can think for themselves. The neuron computer works in a way similar to the human brain, although much simplified according to the textbook The Computer Continuum.

You will find on the computer ergonomic products, accessories, equipment, injuries, safety products and allow customization of your work site to a new level. Just click in search mode on your computer screen, type in keyboards and you will get 20,000 hits or more. Where are the reputable keyboards and keypads found? In the rest of this chapter, I will discuss and name significant products and ideas given on alternative keyboards and devices used to replace standard keyboard use. TIFAQ.com articles include general information, ergonomics, organizations, services and also those who resell these items. They include software, accessories and other products, pointing devices, speech recognition and alternative keyboards as Furniture.

## RESOURCES

There are forums for questions about RSI and ERGO, support groups and related links. This web site is provided by the CTD Resource Network, links. The site contains "a wide variety of information about repetitive strain injuries (RSI's), resources for dealing with these ailments and a broad description of assistive products to reduce injury risk and symptoms." There are keyboard users that have developed both right and left handed injuries and are unable to use their hands and arms. Voice recognition systems have been developed. These are very slow systems. They are getting better. Many professionals are using these just to relieve the hands and fingers. With the use of a microphone they can stand up and move around getting a bit of a mini break in the days routine of sitting at the work station. Foot pedals systems have also been developed to accomplish the same for these keyboard users with both hand injuries. Dragon Naturally Speaking is the system that I set up on my home computer. If you prefer to read about voice systems first, the book by Dan Newman, Talk to Your Computer, is a reference. Newman states you can dictate to your PC at 100 words per minute, even if you can't type, find the system that's right for you, send email and surf the Web by voice and free your hands from keyboard stress.

There are professional and basic editions for voice systems. Prices range from $50.00 to $700.00. Other systems are IBM ViaVoice Basic and ViaVoice Pro. Commercial programs are available too to help corporations and individuals for ergonomic training. Many of these programs are developed by medical professionals. Ergo Health from CorpMed, LLC can be reviewed at their website. This program was written by an Occupation Physician. This is an online office ergo training program.

ErgoSmart is produced by Datachem Software, Inc., the price $695.00 estimated. This is a "low cost, self-paced, interactive and easy-to-use software training tool that teaches your employees how to work comfortably with their computers." The program is used "in more than 400 different organizations worldwide." ErgoTips "allows you to easily make an unlimited number of copies than can be installed on every stand alone computer at your site" for an estimated "$495.00." They claim they are "now licensed for use by over One Quarter Million users in more than 200 sites worldwide."

David Brown, in Australia, has developed an ergonomics training and self-help software program with approximate cost, $5.00 per user. His Road to Comfort program has "been translated into more than 27 languages, and over half a million licensed copies have been printed by IBM, the New Zealand Government and Ericsson Computers, universities, workers compensation insurers, and government bodies." "This ergonomics training software covers workstation adjustment, remedying discomfort, workplace exercises, stress, and workplace relationships." David Brown believes you must "find a balance between corporate responsibility and individual responsibility for health in the workplace." I certainly agree with his premise.

Ergosaver, Inc. developed a program for $25.00 and "uses the Scandinavian training method: highly personalized, focused, results-oriented and fun experiences to maximize well-being and long-term benefits while improving productivity." In addition to "musculoskeletal disorders, repetitive stress injuries, carpal tunnel syndrome", the program mentions other discomforts associated with PC use." "Backaches, headaches and eye strain" are included. This program "integrates the efforts of in-house or external ergonomists and safety managers." Now I know why I keep Visine at my computer table. In England, Infinite Innovations Ltd. has developed ScreamSaver, "which can be customized to each individual's needs to combat the many problems with using a computer for a long period of time." "Users can use ScreamSaver to prompt them to take breaks" in different time frames which can be set or fixed. This program states there are computer problems with RSI, back and neck pain, eye strain and headaches, temporary myopia and stress. The list of computer related problems is getting longer and longer. RestReminder "simply reminds you when it is the time to rest." You may obtain a "free 30 day trial" "tool to prevent RSI or carpal tunnel syndrome." Alen Jevsenak has written a program "fit@work" and a free demo is available at their website http://www.fitatwork.com. This "animated virtual instructor takes care of your health and keeps you fit-at-work" which "directs you regularly to short and varying exercise breaks."

ErgoSentry "can pay for itself in several areas many times over" by lowering insurance and healthcare costs. They believe that "poorly setup workstations or postures slowly damage the soft tissues of your hands, wrists, and arms causing RSI damage." They advocate "to not ignore your symptoms of RSI and the pain is very real and the disability can be permanent." This may be the time to start a journal of the discomfort you have while at your work station. Be sure and include, the time, the date, what you are working on when the symptoms start. Micronite developed the A.R.M.S. (Avoid Repetitive Motion Syndrome) with an estimated price of $39.95 or the deluxe price and program for $79.95 which logs computer activity. This program offers both an exercise manager and digital video with exercises. Other commercial programs at the TIFAQ website are WorkPace, no only monitors all mouse and keyboard usage but a customized break regime. Dr. Wigley and Dr. Turner, both from New Zealand, offer a one-month trial version for a free workpace.com download at their website.

All of these commercial programs note rest breaks and exercises as essential components for long term computer use. StretchBreak state in their program written by health care professionals "over 75% of all workers compensation claims relate to RSI" and if "you expect to be healthy", "you need a stretch break" using "Power-Pause." If you use a laptop most of the time, there are reclinable laptop stands available from Keynamics LLC.

The kinesis-ergo.com/savant website 20 key offers the PS/2 model requiring "no software and has a built-in pass through connection" for your PS/2 keyboard. For the USB model, drivers (provided) are required for re-programming. For either model, you "program the keypad by typing on your keyboard the key actions." "To program the PS/2keypad simply attach a PS/2 keyboard and set the rotary "play/program" selector." The price stated "$129.00." Look closely at the prices because tigerdirect.com/applications "offer for #89.95 a 20 key programmable keypad, USB." This keypad will "reduce complex and repetitive keyboard tasks to a single keystroke." It may be at your place of work, a complicated system and require custom input devices. This you can find at laube.com/products. As many changes are made daily in types of PS/2 devices, compare what is in the internet information and in your control panel.

For more information about keypads, the website digikey.com or you can go to electroneamericas.com. For standard keypad information go to globalspec.com. There are 86 companies that make standard keypads and 27 companies who make programmable keypads. Another company that produces mouse and trackballs is ergoguys.com. Earlier I mentioned Fentek Industries in the USA and Maltron in the UK who make left handed keyboards and other assistive products.

After you assess your computer workstation and your directionality needs, it may be easy to buy one of those and a simple keypad input device for the right side. But, look at all models before you buy from the Internet or go to an electronics store. Go armed with your new knowledge and select the best input devices based on your dominance which is coming up in the chapter on Dexterity Training.

For those injured workers with mouse connected injuries, the roller ball mouse was developed. Many workers have moved the mouse to the left hand side of the keyboard. Mouses or mice, if you prefer, can be purchased with the clicker on the left or the right, to account for your handedness. But which one to select while in the store? Be patient, we are getting to that part of the book. According to Stan Miastkowski, special to PC World technology magazine, the lead sentence "Microsoft Mouse Frees Lefties." For $54.95 you can buy their IntelliMouse as an optical sensor to work as an ambidextrous pointing device. Miastkowski agrees with me there is more than bias in this world of dominant right handed individuals. This sensor has five programmable buttons and can be used with either Universal Serial PS/2 mouse ports. Again, you must check with the options on your computer and compare with what is being offered to date.

At the time of this 2009 writing, the second study of IRS workers is underway. According to Dr. Naomi Swanson, "We are interested in determining whether *ergonomic* computer mice designs are useful in preventing or alleviating musculoskeletal problems. Study participants have been assigned to one of six ergonomic mouse conditions, a placebo mouse condition, or a conventional mouse condition, and are using their assigned mouse for a year. We are periodically collecting musculoskeletal symptom and other data from them, as well as physical exam information at the beginning and end of the study."

Microsoft has the WheelMouse Optical USB/PS2 for your ergonomic fit, left or right handed, and requires 128 MB, Model D6600052. More options for pointing devices are MicroPoint Pro by Altra. This is an easy-to-use mouse scrolling system. Eye Control Technologies, Inc. offers "precise cursor control through simple head movement allowing your hands to remain on your keyboard, or at your side." Estimated price is $99.00. At a much higher price of $2495.00 from EyeTech Digital Systems, LLC "provides an efficient alternative to the mouse. It moves the cursor according to the user's eye movements." Quick Glance "has complete accessibility to all Windows features-without lifting a finger." "Voice dictation software can also be used with the Quick Glance system." Gyration, Inc. makes GyroMouse Pro and "is the only cordless mouse you can use on or off the desktop." By simply picking up the mouse "it automatically tracks your hand movement, guiding the cursor accordingly" and has a "range of 40 feet."

Origin Instruments Corp. developed the HeadMouse for Desktops & Portables for a cost of $1695.00. This sensor program "replaces the standard desktop computer mouse for people who cannot use their hands." This device "translates movements of a user's head into directly proportional movements of the computer mouse pointer." "A remote switch interface is available for wireless transfer of adaptive switch inputs from a wheelchair to the computer." Wow? HeadMaster Plus "is a head pointing system that takes the place of a mouse." "Just move your head and the mouse cursor moves on the screen. Puff on the tube to make selection."

With this system, you "can change from Apple to IBM compatibility just by flipping a switch." Their cost, $995.00.

NOHANDS Mouse "eliminates stress on the delicate hand-wrist area by moving mouse control to the feet." You "can have complete control of the cursor without having to take your hands off the keyboard or your eyes off the monitor." We know from artists calendars marketed that great artwork has been made by the disabled with use of their feet and not their hands. Chat rooms can be good or can be bad; you just need to make sure you want a response. One website, CNET Community Letter wrote in 2005 that "Computer related injuries are no laughing matter." One write in stated his "initial mouse substitute was a touchpad and it eliminated most of the wrist and arm movement." He "worked with the Cirque mouse but its movement was not sensitive enough for graphics work." He researched about mice and "found that the key attribute to my mouse alternatives was to avoid having the hand in the extended palm-down position, so the forearm would not be rotated." With that in mind, he "tried the Renaissance Mouse, now provided by 3M." "It comes in two sizes, depending on your hand width." Then he moved to the "Evoluent Vertical Mouse 2." He is certainly trying to be the best he can be by trying out different mice to do his job better and reduce his chance of work injury.

In the November 22, 2007 web site announcement by PC Joint, the MultiTouch 2.0 comes to Apple computers (described in a new patent application) for their small input devices like iPhone or iPod Touch. In Apple's own words the identification and classification of intuitive hand configurations and motions enables unprecedented integration of typing, resting, scrolling, 3D manipulation, and handwriting into a versatile, ergonomic computer input device. With this product you could track and recognize all the movements of your hands and fingers on or near the touch surface. Another 2008 mouse entry is the vibrating mouse. This is a mouse "that vibrates" according to the Dec. 27, 2007 Science Daily News. These are some of the kinds of newfangled ergonomic products that Alan Hedge, International authority on office ergonomics, studies to see if they can prevent repetitive motion injuries. Hedge estimated 100 million people now use computers in the United States. "One-third to one-half of all compensatory injuries are repetitive-motion injuries associated with office-type work", says Hedge, professor of design and environmental analysis in Cornell's College of Human Ecology. The market continues to develop products as shown at the 2008 Computer Electronics Show in Las Vegas, Nevada. The addition of a Bracelet Mouse for the wrist and a Ring Mouse for your pointer finger by Globlink Technology, Inc. is advertised as the "innovative smallest Mouse." This company also makes the wireless keypads with an optical trackball for keypads, left or right or right to left.

EyerCise was developed "that breaks up your day with periodic sets of stretches and visual training exercises. The stretches work all parts of your body, relieving tension and helping prevent RSI" and "eye strain." The premise of this "warns you to take breaks after a configurable interval." It interrupts "you based on clock time rather than typing time." Izquierdo JC et al. in their 2004 Puerto Rico medical study Factors Leading to the Computer Vision Syndrome: an issue at the contemporary workplace believes vision and eye related problems are common among users. These researchers concluded their findings show that most important factor leading to the syndrome is the angle gaze at the computer monitor.

In a conversation with Optometrist Annette Brabham in February 2005, she too believes in this syndrome and while tending to her patients, inquires about computer usage and reminds her patients, you need to look slightly downward at your computer screen to reduce the problem according to both eye specialists in ergonomic education, pain is diminished in computer users when gazing downward at angles of 14 degrees or more.

Time spent at the computer monitor will change the organ of

sight or vision. Some functional changes in the eye can be pointed out. A Russian study in 2004 showed dramatic changes from the first hour to the second hour. So time on task in computer users and eyes effects declining tear production. No authors were listed in this article. Texas Industrial Peripherals developed HulaPoint which "combines the features of a trackball and a joystick for a truly user friendly experience" with an innovative three button design. And there is the Graphire2, which is a "pressure sensitive pen & cordless, batteryless mouse." The pen operates on finger pressure levels and "has no ball to clean so it never skips." In this past year, Fentek Industries developed a keyboard for left handers with several variations for both PC and Mac users. Developers in keyboard and keypad design know we have a problem.

What is basically different about all the new designs of keyboards? The majority are attempts to change work postures. At the NIOSH web site, 1/ split and rotated keyboard with wrist rests, 2/ split and tented keyboard , 3/ adjustable negative slope, 4/ concave well keyboard, 5/ curved keyboard are just some of the names. The alternative keyboards have been shown to promote neutral wrist posture. Numerical pad developments are also being made but these are not of the likeness of the original keyboard and new learning will be required to operate those. Their web site is fentek-ind.com and from review of the picture at the web site, it appears the numerical portion was just moved to the opposite side in 2002. Then, in 2003, from my observation, Fentek added a mirror image pad but no other information.

For your workers who are disabled Adaptive Technology that Provides Access to Computers is from the U. S. Department of Education (ERIC). Whether blindness, low vision, hearing or speech impairments, specific learning disabilities or mobility, help is available by calling RESNA in your state or another contact is the DO-IT program at the University of Washington from their funding by the National Science Foundation. Which one would you select while you are reviewing their web site?

Again, we are moving in that direction of determining how to select computer devices based on your dominance. If you have looked closely at the cost of many of these peripherals devices, the costs range from $5.00 to over $3000.00.If you receive many phone calls in your normal work day, I hope you have a headset. The basic Platonic headset uses the microphone and speaker plugs on your PC. Their models have a behind-the-neck style of bracket and the cost is $20.00. A website devoted to helping RSI and computer users is the DMOZ website. They offer "culling out the bad and useless (information) and keeping only the best information about RSI."

The information found in this book will save you money, time and help you and those who work with you, preventing work related computer injuries. There are many more attempts by companies trying to rectify the design of the keyboard and keypads. Try going to any large electronic computer store (Frys, Office Depot, Office Max, Circuit City, CompUSA, Best Buy) and you will find many variations of new ergonomic solutions for computer work stations. Again, I ask, how do you know what to buy? The store clerks can show you what is in stock, on the shelf or can order. But they cannot assess your handedness between the hands or fingers

Before the end of this book, you will be comfortable knowing more in advance when you select or recommend keyboards, keypads and other devices for your ergonomic solutions. One easy place I have found to purchase accessories is the PC Connection catalog which can offer everything in overnight delivery, if they have it in stock. The website is pcconnection.com.

Repetitive Motion Injuries result in the longest work absences and Days Away From Work from Carpal Tunnel Syndrome from the Monthly Labor Review, a U. S. Dept. of Labor website, bls.gov. By reviewing closely the types of remedies developed from these inventors and companies, cost involved, you will see why there is so much negativity at the workstation which should spur you to take a critical look at your computer workstation. Also you can put it in the back of your mind, what purchases you may need to be looking at as you progress through this book.

One of the premises by reading this book is, you will save money by not buying what you do not need. Review the Purchasing Checklist that you downloaded from the OSHA eTool website.

# CHAPTER FIVE

*Wisdom is perishable. Unlike information or knowledge, it cannot be stored in a computer or recorded in a book. It expires with each passing generation.*

**Sid Taylor**

## BACKGROUND INFORMATION

In an article by Brad A. Myers's A Brief History of Human Computer Interaction Technology, he summarizes the historical development of major advances in human-computer interaction technology, emphasizing the pivotal role of university research in the advancement of the field. Many of the computer electronic companies use higher learning such as the Human Computer Interaction Institute at Carnegie Mellon University for their research although there are private companies like Forrester Research who have developed innovative solutions with computer systems for people with disabilities.

Much of the information that has been presented thus far is from companies, developers of hardware and software and our government. As we move through the chapters, you will listen and read the words of notable computer experts that give you their knowledge and experience with their overviews comparing the inner workings of the computer with their hardware and software to the inner working of the brain, as they understand it. Later you will see the more respected medical and educational literature from our National Institute of Health (NIH) and the National Library of

Medicine (NLM). My plan and I hope your plan; you will be able to see how your computer and you are connected and to show why you need to make changes at your workstation. Then, create your options for transforming your workstation to use both hands in different ways to increase your productivity and longevity using your computer with my training method.

Review of recent and pertinent literature will provide us with the details needed to train your left hand for numerical data entry with the steps needed for the process. This will be especially useful for those readers who wish to know the how and why they are doing something different or for the teacher who has a need for learning how to train the non-preferred hand in a motor task. Or, then again, for training leaders in safety and risk management and/or case managers who are seeking ways to return their injured workers to their job or the job market.

You may or may not have at this time an injury from over use but after you read this part of the book, you may choose to use this knowledge yourself or share the information with someone you know who is having this type of problem. The end result of this review with training will focus on modifying work practices of computer /keypad users to prevent overuse injury by reducing the number of repetitions of the hands/fingers/arms. Regardless of type of numerical input device, alternating activity between the right hand and left hand will reduce the load on the right hand during tasks using the usual computer and numerical keypad or the computer with a stand alone numerical input device.

Recent research has shown new patterns of coordination can be learned. You have only to look at the new computer games that require use of both hands. And to carry this thought further, using the entire computer work station with numerous devices attached requiring use of both hands in a coordinated manner. A Telephonic Nurse Case Manager, like me, at her desk, manages claims from a telephone with ear piece at the computer workstation requiring a coordinated effort and they have a risk, along of course with their Claims Adjuster counterpart.

Other people also at risk for these injuries are keyboard operators and computer specialists and secretaries or from office worker employees. Also new mothers, women between the ages of 40–60 due to hormonal changes, obesity, thyroid disorders, diabetes, gout or arthritis are easy targets for CTS or MSD.

## NAME OF DIAGNOSIS FOR COMPUTER RELATED INJURIES

The diagnosis for hand overload injuries is often Carpal Tunnel Syndrome (CTS), repetitive stress (RSI) and tendonitis or tenosynovitis due to the frequency of finger/wrist movements. Often degeneration of the cranial vertebrae or brachial plexus injuries leads to these types of complaints. Research categories reviewed in this section of the book are anatomy and physiology and brain organization. Later, hand and finger movements, musicians, tactile objects (touch) discrimination, motor dominance, circling tasks, gender, performance, individual differences, old learning and new learning, training and education, left to right directionality, similar studies, musculoskeletal disorders and injury prevention will be presented to you. Finally, a summary of expectations and recommendations for learning how to use the numeric keypad and mouse with your non- preferred hand.

Preventing the onset of cumulative trauma injuries within an office environment brings many potential benefits for employers in terms of direct and indirect cost savings. The key point for prevention is striving to reduce the number of repetitions. According to a study by Travers et al. (2002) of office workers and VDT, "a trend in symptom otology was identified, whereby symptoms appeared to increase as duration of VDT exposure increased." This is time on the job task for computer users. Three/fifths of all occupational injuries can be attributed to various debilitating hand and wrist disorders according to The John Marshall Journal of Computer and Information Law. "Without reliable medical or scientific evidence showing a relationship between use and injury, the question arises, is it necessary for computer manufacturers to begin placing warnings on their keyboards which urge users to pay more attention to safety and comfort?"

According to OSHA in their eTool website, "alternative left hand keyboards which have the keypad permanently affixed to the left side of the keyboard are available as are keyboards with a detached keypad. These allow the user to switch positions for either left or right hand use." Also "programmable stand alone keypads are available which can be programmed to facilitate either right or left hand usage" as possible solutions. But "this arrangement can be limiting to the left handed workers or right handed workers who are recovering from injury and are attempting to remain functional during recovery." There is more to left hand usage and the reason for this book and training method.

## TWO DIRECTION TYPES

Numeric keypads are used for data entry by banks, credit card companies, financial management institutions and health care companies. Robin High at the University of Oregon, Statistical Programmer and Consultant states data entry can be a very laborious, and often a very boring task, prone to errors resulting from fatigue or carelessness. With those facts in mind, after a presentation by me at the DFAS Comptrollers monthly meeting in Northwest Florida at the Pensacola Naval Air Station in July 2005, these were the questions asked and results. As a result of this presentation, would you consider?

• Daily warm up exercises to help prevent computer related injury?
• Completing numerical data entry training with the left hand?
• Completing mouse training with the left hand?

- Using a dual numerical keyboard/keypad?
- Are you right handed, left handed or mixed hander?
- Do you have any symptoms of CTS?
- How long have you worked in accounting?

After the handwriting test and finger circling test, are you? Mirrored in both hands and fingers or Parallel or? Yes or No?

## ANALYSIS OF ASMC SEMINAR (ACCOUNTANTS, FINANCE, AUDITING COMPTROLLERSHIP GROUP)

- 23 responders were from the When Left is Right presentation.
- 100% would use a daily warm up exercise program to prevent computer related injuries.
- Responders had 5–32 years working with numerical data entry.
- 78% would try the mouse training with the left hand.
- 69% would try the numerical data keypad training with the left hand and two responders stated already do left hand keypad and one stated would try right.
- 69% would try the dual keyboard/keypad.
- Of this group, 69% were right handed, 21% left handed and 8% mixed handed.
- Of the responders, 47% had hand and finger complaints and 1 shoulder complaint of pain.
- Of the responders, 39% were mirror/mirror image, 26% were parallel/parallel image, and 34% had different mirror/parallel image or parallel/mirror image results.

Why are these percentages impressive? The overwhelming interest in prevention of computer related problems with a daily warm-up exercise and what types of exercise to use during breaks and rest time at work or at home. The majority of these workers use a computer at work and at home. From my research, I knew we would have a certain number of mixed handers and left handers. I also knew for sure just because you were trained by your right hand with the numbers going left to right on the keypad that you could very well be different in the selection of a keypad for left hand use. In other words, for the left hand, left to right or right to left direction of the numbers?

Accuracy is likely to suffer when you're attempting to manually enter data from a data source directly into a computer file. A primary rule of data entry is that it should never be done with a word processing program. Various specialized programs are available for data entry that is far more appropriate according to Dr. High. Ainsworth at qwerty.com has a patent describing his development of two-handed input systems with his approach to eliminate carpal tunnel and other RSI problems. But, this does not mention any interference in the neural network of the fingers in his Ainsworth Keypad Trainer software program. Ainsworth states you can use either hand for the same device just by positioning the keyboard with keypad. But this does not account for our USA culture for reading sequentially left to right and then transposing that old learning to new learning of the non preferred hand.

Due to human factors and brain organization this sequential learning for the non preferred hand will either be parallel sequencing or mirror image sequencing based upon the person's dominance. More about this will be explained in the chapters outlining the establishment of your directionality and research about how the brain is organized. What better way to start than by going to one of the pioneers in the computer industry.

## INTERVIEW WITH A RETIRED IBM EXECUTIVE

What a wonderful afternoon I had interviewing John Hipp, a retired IBM research executive. We discussed computer networking and human brain networking for starters.

*Grafton:* Where do you see the next level of computers?

*Hipp:* Whoever can put the largest amount of memory in a chip will be the winner. Just look at what happened in the 50s. First the 700 series followed by the Stretch Computer. Its goal was to shoot for the stars, but we only made it to the moon, therefore this computer was discarded. Then followed the System 360 series with the Model 50 being 'my baby'. The Stretch Computer was magnificent.

*Grafton:* When you were at IBM, how was carpal tunnel syndrome handled?

*Hipp:* I had it myself. I learned early when the pain starts in your forearms, you need to stop. Rest your hands: shake them out, stretch out your fingers and hands. When you look at Carpal Tunnel Syndrome, you have not only to bear the pain and the agony but also, work productivity goes down and that affects the bottom line in corporations. When you look at computer users, many have had to move on to other jobs. Programmers are especially vulnerable to the problem.

*Grafton:* What do you think of the proposed title of my book?

*Hipp:* Computer companies need to find the left handers. With your idea of training the left hand when everything is made for the right hander, immediate success in the computer world for the left hander will follow.

*Grafton:* I want you to take the two simple experiments for determining finger directionality between the two hands

*Hipp:* OK

*Grafton:* Now that you know you are 'mirrored', what do you think about the dual numerical keyboard and keypad?

*Hipp:* That's a great idea and you know what else? You need to let corporate executives know you can increase productivity with your left handers. So many programmers are left handed but keyboards are made for the right hander.

*Grafton:* A study was done at the University of Toronto which concluded it takes 2 weeks to train yourself to use the mouse on the left side but no mention of where the clicker should be or programmed to be. What do you know about mouse injuries?

*Hipp:* If there is anything that needs changing right away, it is the mouse. Again, they are made for the right hander. If there is anything you need to add in your book, if you are hiring a programmer, hire a left hander and train him using your idea. In other words, look for the left hander; they will be successful right away.

And then a rebuttal comes from computer programmer Mathew Monroe who writes computer games software.

*Grafton:* What is there you disagree with?

*Monroe:* Mouses nowadays are programmable and are easy to use with either hand. This is what allowed me to teach myself to use my left hand. The piece of hardware that needs to be changed is the keyboard. As this is where the stress comes on the hands due to having to hold them over the keys at an awkward angle and repeat many of the same strokes over and over. With the mouse you can rest your wrist on the mouse pad with a gel wrist pad. This gel pad maintains the correct angle for your wrist at all times and allows you to rest your wrist. The keyboard on the other hand, because of its layout makes use of a gel pad ineffective. This is what needs changing.

*Grafton:* What do you see next in computer technology?

*Monroe:* I know what I want to see come down the technology pipeline and that is a better keyboard, or alternative for the keyboard.

*Grafton:* What about my idea of the dual computer keyboard?

*Monroe:* Programmers are pushed to produce, so the idea of the dual numerical keyboard and keypad would be a boon for the employee and the employer.

In the Game Room section of the "Ft. Walton Beach newspaper, January 4, 2005 edition, Playing games fun; programming not" is the lead. An "employee who posted a Web log on the working conditions her husband endures that has generated heated buzz throughout the gaming community." At the website, usabilitymustdie.com, writer Frank Lynch asked "A left-handed keyboard? How I've longed for an enter key on the left side." Computer users are asking or help in the design of keyboards and keypads for everyone, not just for right handers.

There are differing numbers given for right handers, left handers and mixed handers but it is expected by this writer that 75–80% of computer users are right handed and 15–20% are a combination of left handers and mixed handers. This 20% group is expected to have a higher performance rate of learning during training using the left hand. The regular standard keyboard/keypad was developed for right handers or left handers who had the ability to become a right hander. The difference in rates is due to a more permissive parental society in learning to use the hands early in life.

## THE COMPUTER WORKSTATION

"There are many right handed programmable keypad options on the market today that enable" "flexibility for data entry" and/or standard keyboards with the keypad on the left side for left handers. Of interest to this researcher is to find a product design that fits human capacities (for you and me) and will allow dual use of the numeric keypad for both the right hand and the left hand.

So far, in Part One, I have given you education in your computer workstation, devices available for purchase, what type of treatment is given for the numerous diagnosis of computer related complaints, what factors you should consider and some alternative solutions. Now, we will bring in the foundation of your learning experience with the exercises needed to reduce or prevent further hand and finger injuries. Plus two simple case histories that explain how a work injury claim progresses from start to finish.

# CHAPTER SIX

*Man is a slow, sloppy and brilliant thinker; the machine is fast, accurate and stupid.*

**William M. Kelly**

## CASE HISTORIES

I first began to work with Worker's Compensation injuries in Las Vegas in 1992 in a rehabilitation facility, then for the Clark County in Las Vegas followed by an international insurance company also in Las Vegas, where I began to manage many hand injury claims. With a summary of actual cases you will begin to see the relationship of the factors leading to injuries and the filing of claims for compensation.

While working in Atlanta as the designated Nurse Case Manager for an international insurance company, I provided medical management on worker injury claims. Of significant interest to me were the clients whose employees utilized computers and numeric keypads such as banks, insurance, credit card, and health care companies. As the designated nurse assigned to one large series of banks for the state of Georgia and a smaller different series of banks in Alabama, one of my jobs was to work with the claims manager, the employer, the physician and therapists to help return these clients to work. Many of the injuries at the banks were due to overuse of the hands and arms. Over use injuries resulted in worker's compensation claims, time off, and lowered productivity by injured workers.

Now that I have introduced you to the disorders found in work injuries with use of the computer and factors that must be considered with some of the alternative solutions, I believe it is appropriate for me to mention a variety of actual claims. Every claim is different because people are different, companies are different and medical providers are different. Another important difference: State Worker's Compensation Laws. Cooperativeness is expected from injured workers with claims but that is not always the case.

## CASE #1, OFFICE WORKER

A difficult case for me follows as a Telephonic Nurse Case Manager, working in Las Vegas, and managing claims also of claimants in California and Utah.

This 45 year old female, office worker was referred to me as she "out of work." The claimant frequently hung up on me when I tried to interview to find out her medical history. The employer reported frequently she did not show up for work, restricted duty, and even missed her doctor appointments. claimant finally told me, after I asked about her history of taking Prednisone, that she was treated 15 years ago for Lupus, but was over that and had not been treated for over 10 years. The occupational doctor requested a referral to a Rheumatologist. I arranged for her to be seen by a specialist more than 50 miles away to determine if her problems with her hands and arms were work related or from long term lupus treatment or lack of follow up treatment. The rheumatology specialist's report revealed he believed her arm and hand problems were not work related but the disease process of Lupus.

## CASE #2, OFFICE WORKER

After receiving a referral from the adjuster for an office worker, we spoke briefly about the new claim from a glass company. The employer told the adjuster, the injured worker had done the same computer job for a long time. Due to her (injured worker) right hand problem, she was now using only one hand (the left) to key in the numbers, no work had been missed and did not see a problem with the claim. I completed a chart review. From review, the diagnosis was wrist tenosynovitis. The treatment plan was for Ibuprofen daily and to discontinue Naproxen, to continue the plan with her previous physical therapy schedule and modified duty at work consisting of limited use of the right hand with left hand typing only. The physical therapy treatment consisted of iontophoresis pads, hot/cold packs, ultrasound and home management training. After speaking with the employer, I found what the claimant's job requirements were. Her job title was a Glass Coordinator with her duties: computer keyboarding. I asked for a copy of her job description but the employer responded they do not have them. I agreed to fax a copy of how to develop a description and employer agreed to do that. I wanted to know how many hours of the day were required on the computer or any other duties. The interview with the worker was conducted by telephone while she was at work. She had worked for the same company and doing the same job for five years.

The injury happened, she explained "when she does a lot of data entry all at once; her right hand swelled up and has pain, numbness and tingling and sometimes the middle and index finger too." According to her, "the therapy was helping and was taking her medication and using a right hand splint with metal." She also said "the physical therapist came out to see her work set up yesterday. She had two work station set ups but the therapist moved things around to where she only has one now." She also said the "Safety Corporate Officer was there this a.m. and he made some suggestions too. He gave her two web sites to review, TIFAQ and Fentek (my communication was working) for ergonomic information, different types of keyboards", etc. The office worker said "keying a lot makes it worse." "She must watch how much she works. At night her pain affects her sleep sometimes." Her responsibilities were "to key data using both hands, but now she is using the left hand as much as possible." She is right handed, 5'8", 183# and is 24 years old. She had missed only one day of work so far. She agreed that she "understood what *light duty* is and agreed to follow doctor's orders" and would call me if any problems. I anticipated her time with length of disability (LOD) would be one month minimum. The employer called and reported "released from the doctor." The claimant reported to me "therapy and the work station changes worked for her." The claims manager reported "she was discharged from the MD after five weeks of treatment" and we agreed I would close my part of the claim.

This was a good outcome for her and for me with a very cooperative injured worker. The education I gave to the adjuster about keyboard injuries, who in turn provided education for the company, decreased the duration of the injury. This is cost containment in health care. A Nurse Case Manager must plan for this when the case is opened and identify when closed. In other words, what effect did my handling of the claim have upon the employee, the employer and the costs associated with the claim? Also I wish to point out; excessive or repetitive use of the keypad appeared to be the problem or cause of the injury. More importantly, this was the claim which caused me to re-think left hand usage and use of the keypads at the keyboard.

# PART THREE

## FOLLOW THE
## RIGHT ROAD

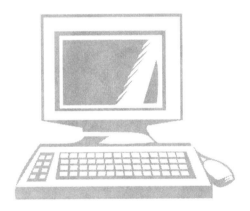

# CHAPTER SEVEN

*Control over computing belongs with users.*

**Brandt Allen**

## THE EXERCISES

If and when you seek medical advice or treatment for a work related injury from a medical office, you will bring back to your employer a work slip. This slip will usually give the diagnosis, what type of work limitations you may have, when your next appointment is, or any treatment or medications recommended which will need to be approved by the employer. If you are injured or having problems with your hands, try to understand the diagnosis names of the muscles and tendons and where they are. Also, when you leave your medical officer's office, collect a copy of all documents for yourself placing them in a folder. You may need them.

## TYPES OF WORKSTATION EXERCISES

In the review of physical exercises recommended for VDT operators by Lee (1992), these researchers "reviewed 127 individual exercises and were analyzed for their suitability for performance in VDT workplaces." "Over one third of the exercises were conspicuous and potentially embarrassing to perform, and half would significantly disrupt the work routine." This study with their "findings suggest a need for greater attention to both the practical and the therapeutic aspects of exercises promoted for VDT users." Disrupting the work routine is not something the employer is willing to do.

For example, in the review of NIOSH research findings "of relevance to 40,000 employees of the Internal Revenue Service and millions of workers in similar work operations, determined the use of a regimen of hourly brief rest breaks reduced musculoskeletal disorders without loss of productivity." This study was done over ten years ago.

## PRODUCTS ON THE MARKET

In the next few paragraphs you will read and note what entrepreneurs are designing for these types of hand and wrist complaints. For those of you who like gadgets, the Flextend Solution may be of interest to assist with the exercises. You can "purchase the Flex Tend glove for 3 monthly payments of $28.00." But, use your ingenuity with a rubber band with no cost to you, just your time. I caution against using any weight training, just use gentle stretching with your hands, wrists and arms. You may not know of the risk of hand sports injuries of weight lifters, tennis and golf enthusiasts (tennis and golf elbow).

For hand, wrist and elbow exercises, this simple group of exercises permits major joints to gradually regain their full range if you have been having problems. What is recommended are five to six repetitions throughout the day consisting of Fist Flexion (make a fist), open and closing of the hand with the thumb (stretch out all fingers), Thumb Extension (close the fingers and stretch the thumb), Flexion and Wrist and Elbow movements (up, down, left, right). You should not feel pain or any increase in swelling during exercise. If you have had surgery on your hand or fingers or therapy from a PT or an OT, you probably already have done those exercises. The downloads that I developed for myself, for my own longevity with computer work, are divided by warm-up while your computer is loading and one for rest breaks. I put them on my desk top. If you are seeing a therapist, show them this book.

The same movements are made by the wrists. When the wrist is in neutral it is neither flexed nor extended, it is straight. By flexing, bend toward the underside of the forearm. By extending, bend toward the upper side of the forearm, as in hitting a tennis forehand drive. Radial flexion in the wrist is neutral but bends flexions toward the thumb, as in tennis during the backhand drive or throwing a Frisbee.

Ulnar flexion too, is placing the wrist in neutral position and bends flexion toward the 5th finger. You may refer to these flexions as curls, i.e. wrist curl.

In an interview with Naturopathic Physician Delores Mangels, from Jacksonville, Florida, I asked her pertinent questions about upper arm exercise with her recommendations for any additional other than those mentioned.

*Grafton:* When did you first hear about Carpal Tunnel Syndrome?

*Mangels:* What I recall are bicyclists, weight lifters especially when triathlon athletes were acquiring sports injuries. But even earlier, waitresses and housekeepers developed these types of disorders.

*Grafton:* Are there particular references you use in your practice?

*Mangels:* The exercise book by Pete Egosure is very good about being pain free. He believes a computer does not have to hurt if you will do his exercises. Circumduction of all of your joints is good. Do not type from the fingers only, type with your shoulder

*Grafton:* You have reviewed the hand and finger exercises. What more would you add for those ailing in the arms?

*Mangels:* When I look and hear what my patient is saying, for example, my left side hurts then you start on the right side. It is the theory of the reflex arc, the opposite side of the body controls the other. You use opposing side exercises. Stretching is good. For pain, use a paraffin bath or heat or soaking in warm water. But if you have swelling, do not use heat. You also need to work (exercise) the arm and shoulder. The wash cloth stretch is good. You do this daily after bathing or showering using your towel. Hold your right arm high holding the towel, drape across your back, holding the left other edge of the towel with your left hand and move the towel sideways up and own. The rhomboid (mid back) muscles are the beginning of your arms and start at the shoulder. If you have pain in that area, you need to release the rhomboids first. Use the body curl in your computer chair to help with your back. One other exercise I use is the wall clock. Put your toes together, stand tall against a wall, hold your arms up high and rotate the opposite you would use on your computer. Consciously use more of your shoulders while typing and that will assist the muscles of the hand, wrist and forearm by pulling in the upper back and shoulder muscles. If you are using a wrist brace, it will shift your problem to the elbow. (These are the exercises Dr. Mangels recommends for rest breaks. Review the body curl, body side bend and wall clock exercises again).

*Grafton:* Would reflexology be of benefit for these hand computer injuries?

*Mangels:* Yes, if you could find one. Reflexologists are easy to find that work on feet but finding one that can also work on the hands is difficult.

*Grafton:* Do you have any "word" benefits for our readers?

*Mangels:* Yes, function monitors structure and thought is boss. In other words, you can analyze your own body performance by paying close attention to your exercise program.

Dr. Mangels gives us a logical and reasonable explanation from her background in holistic health care. What Dr. Mangels brings into this is how the two sides of the body must work together to have balance. If your body is out of balance, then you need to be rebalanced. Although no research statistics were found to confirm or refute the value or any of these exercises, they have been suggested by various medical providers. What I am recommending are exercises with your hands, fingers and arms: daily warm-up exercises; for use when you are turning on your computer while it is loading and for rest break exercises for your back, arms and shoulders. With practice, you will be able to incorporate the exercises for relief throughout your work day. For example, do not work more than two hours without taking some type of exercise break.

The American Society of Hand Therapists recommend stretching of the of the arms and shoulders, by folding your hands together and turning your palms away and you extend your arms forward, then turn your palms away but this time extend your arms overhead (as explained in the wall clock stretch). By pushing the back of your elbow toward your body across your chest toward the opposite chest is a good stretch too. You can also raise one arm overhead on the bent elbow and of course, stretch both arms. If you are a tennis or baseball player, you know this stretch. Another good stretch is to extend a hand in front of you, bending the hand down toward the floor with one hand, turn the palm up and stretch the hand toward your body.

For simple strengthening exercises: by taking a small rubber band, you can place the rubber band on each finger separately and move each finger through the four muscle movements of the left hand (up, down, left, right) while mildly stretching the rubber band. In using the left hand, most right handers find they can flex the 2nd joint of the middle finger easy. Also flexing the 4th and 5th fingers together at the 2nd joint are considered easy finger movements. Too, keeping the 2nd and 3rd fingers in extension together and separating the 4th and 5th fingers in extension together is also an easy movement. Try this too. Hand strengthening with a rubber ball (you can use a tennis ball) and stretch both hands.

Exercise should not be painful, but if they are, consult your doctor according to the hand therapy organization. Try the side bends stretch while sitting. Take that same view and you can do a simple side neck stretch. These exercises are to be done slowly. For those of you who have the beginning of a forward tilt in your upper body from years of sitting at your desk or workstation, this backward stretch is recommended by Dr. Abe Cardwell (Instructor at the Life Center) in Atlanta, Ga. This sitting backward stretch should be included in the Rest Break exercise portion and used daily. Lean your head back while holding your arms and shoulders behind your back then hold for five seconds.

## ANATOMY AND PHYSIOLOGY AND THE SENSORY MOTOR SYSTEM

Strain and Counter strain is a process which osteopathic physicians use to balance the body. This manipulation technique identifies a point of tenderness which correlates with an area of dysfunction of a joint or a body tissue. What is good about this treatment is it is entirely atraumatic and the patient helps to direct the treatment through feedback with regard to the tenderness. For more information about this technique, go to straincounterstrain.com.

Neuropsychologists have studied the relationship between neural mechanisms and behavior. Their scientific methods are ablation (removing a part of the nervous system), electrical recording and stimulation (EEG), use of the microscope, neuroimaging and the use of chemicals. Let us hope we can change the course of computer users without having to seek help with the sensory and motor nerves. But then again, in nano technology, the sensing from our fingers with their energy may be a forerunner to that science for computer users.

There are two parts to human movement: sensory and motor nerves. In developing their model, Goldberg M. and Casette (1981) reviewed the anatomical literature which shows the right hemisphere of the human brain has more myelinated neurons than the left hemisphere and should, therefore, be capable of more rapid processing. Furthermore, the right hemisphere appears to have more connections to the rest of the brain than the left.

The motor nerves are located in cervical 6, 7, 8 (the neck) and thoracic 1, 3, 4 (upper back). Those are the neck and upper back nerves close to the vertebrae. In his book The Mind, Anthony Smith describes the sensory component of the neural system "Cervical 6: outside (or lateral) forearm, extending as far as the thumb and forefinger. Cervical 7: central forearm to central finger. Cervical 8: inner forearm to part of ring (or third) and little finger. Thoracic 1: inner (or medial) side of upper and lower arm, and remaining areas of third and little (fourth) finger." As you read, trace with your hand and fingers to reinforce your learning. Smith continues his discussion with the cranial motor nerves by stating the muscles controlled by No. 11 (Accessory) lie in the shoulder (such as the trapezius), the arm and the throat. As you read this information, continue to place you hand on the areas mentioned to help with your memory of those body parts. The brachial plexus "is made up of nerves which come out of the middle and lower neck and upper back. After they interconnect, to form the plexus, they branch off to supply different areas, especially the shoulders, arms, elbows, wrists, hands and fingers." According to the Tedd Koren 1997 publication, "Pins and needles in the fingers" are a sign of plexus injury or disorder. Sometimes there is pain and sometimes numbness with this problem. Find the plexis by placing your hand on the opposing side between your breast and your shoulder. Many researchers find there are more neck and back complaints with computer workers than the hands and fingers which is the reason I am asking you to take in this information about the different parts of the body and the body systems.

## CORPUS COLOSSUM AND THE
## TWO SIDES OF THE BRAIN

According to the historical overview of clinical evidence in right brain, left brain research, "motor control and sensory pathways between the brain and the rest of body are almost completely crossed. Each hand is served primarily by the cerebral hemisphere on the opposite side." By placing your left hand on the left side of your brain and moving your right hand. Pause. Then placing your right hand on the right side of your brain and moving your left hand will give you your own overview of how this research applies. The corpus colossum is the major nerve-fiber tract connecting the two sides of the brain. Review the picture in this chapter for the descriptive drawing. Writers and researchers alike discussing dominance, agree "the brain's left half both controls the muscles of and receives sensation from the right hand half of the body. This switch-over, of the left controlling the right and vice versa" is true for most functions." The same agreement the brain's right half both controls the muscles of and receives sensation from the left half of the body. In other words, the movements of human beings are controlled by the brain via the nervous system.

Many structures in animal and human life show left-right asymmetry. Our lungs and kidneys are paired organs and our cerebral

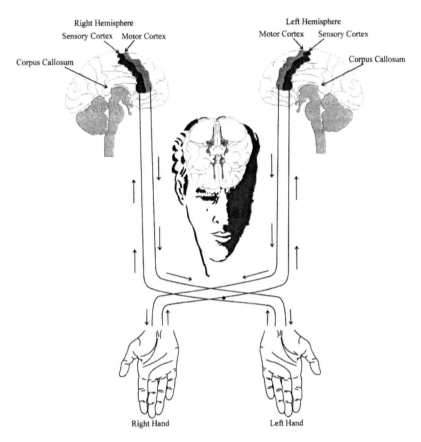

*Right Hand / Hemisphere, Left Hand / Hemisphere /*
*Corpus Colossum*

hemispheres can also be considered as a paired organ. Even monozy-
gotic twin pairs can be found discordant for handedness. Some
show mirror imaging of several features and may be caused by late
twinning, when the original embryo has already lost its bilateral
symmetry. According to Smith, that "touch is everywhere, and is
known as a general, rather than a special, sense. The receptors are
unevenly distributed so there is no uninformative of sensation on
each individual's twenty square feet of skin. On the back there are
fewest, on forearm and legs there are more, on the palms more still"
"and on the fingertips" "most of all."

Springer and Deutsch in their book Left Brain/Right Brain, (two psychologists) state each hemisphere appears to be approximately a mirror image of the other, very much in keeping with the general left right symmetry of the human body. Their theory of control of the body's basic movements and sensations are evenly divided between the two cerebral hemispheres. But they agree that by examining the abilities of our two hands are not equivalent in all respects. Most people have a dominant hand but few people are truly ambidextrous.

In the new book by Malfese and Segalowitz entitled Brain Lateralization in Children, Chapter Ten, by the noted researcher and writer, the Marcel Kinsbourne contribution states "with handedness behavioral control is an issue. It is well known that non-right-handers are not simply mirror-image replicas of the dextral norms." I could not agree with this statement more as I have found with many presentations with feedback from listeners, this is so.

Satz (1972) states that "right-handedness is a genetically determined trait. The puzzle is other right-handers appear to function as well as true right-handers but they are not." There are mirror image and parallel image people with brain organization. Finding out which right-handers are true and which ones are not true (mixed-handers, ambidextrous) is the key to solving this puzzle. My patent gives the answer along with this book. What a concept? Make a right-hander a left-hander at the workstation and the left-hander is happy allowing themselves to function with their true handedness pattern. Porac C. and Coren (1975) asked is eye dominance a part of generalized laterality? Handedness has been the most extensively studied aspect of lateral dominance according to these researchers. "Control of the limbs is basically a function of the contralateral cerebral hemisphere. This may indicate some sort of general cerebral dominance." These researchers summarized their findings and confirm that better consistency is found for right eye dominants than left. In addition, sex differences emerge indicating more consistent eye and limb preferences as well as stronger eye dominance scores in male subjects. This probably culturally conditioned with increased assertiveness in women the male/female difference should decrease.

From pictures and artists drawings in the anatomy and physiology of the human brain, it is far easier to understand the different areas of the motor cortex. But, the motor and somatosenory areas of the cortex are projections of areas of the body. When you look at the face, tongue and fingers, their representations are very large in comparison to others. Starting at the top of the cortex on the left side would be the leg, hip, trunk, neck, head, shoulder, arm, hand, fingers, thumb, eye, nose, face, lips, teeth, tongue, pharynx and abdomen. Just below the face are the foot and genitals. This is the somatosensory cortex explanation. Then, for the motor cortex, toes, ankle, knee, hip, trunk, shoulder, arm, hand, wrist, fingers, thumb, neck, brow, eye, face lips, jaw, tongue and swallowing. The lips take up more space in the motor cortex than they do in the somatosensory cortex, as the lips do more muscle-controlled moving than they do sensing. This explanation is from Brain Function and Blood Flow from Scientific American in 1978. You may wish to re read the last two paragraphs and placing your hand on the areas mentioned.

Recent studies from Byl N. and McKenzie (2000) at the University of California in San Francisco "show that rapid, nearly simultaneous, stereotypical repetitive fine motor movements can degrade the sensory representation of the hand and lead to a loss of normal motor control with a target task, referred to as occupational hand cramps or focal hand dystonia." This particular diagnosis had symptoms of hand cramping. "The purpose of this prospective follow-up study was to determine whether symptomatic patients in jobs demanding high levels of repetition could be relieved of awkward, involuntary hand movements following sensory discriminative retraining complemented by a home program of sensory exercises, plus traditional posture, relaxation, mobilization, and fitness exercises." Twelve patients participated in the study. They all had "occupational hand cramps, as diagnosed by a neurologist. Each patient was evaluated by a trained, independent research assistant before treatment and three to six months after treatment, by use of a battery of sensory, motor, physical, and functional performance tests. Care was provided by a physical therapist or a supervised physical therapist student in an outpatient clinic." These study participants training consisted of "1) heavy schedules of sensory training with and without biofeedback to restore the sensory representation of the hand, and 2) instructions in stress-free hand use, mirror imagery, mental rehearsal, and mental practice techniques designed to stop the abnormal movements and facilitate normal hand control. Patients were instructed in therapeutic exercises to be performed in the home to improve postural alignment, reduce neural tension, facilitate relaxation, and promote cardiopulmonary fitness" (289–301). You may be skeptical about the use of exercise and various treatment modalities but this study certainly supports the methods written in this chapter. "This descriptive study that includes patients with occupation-related focal hand dystonia provides evidence that aggressive sensory discriminative training complemented by traditional fitness exercises to facilitate musculoskeletal health can improve sensory processing and motor control of the hand."

Even Microsoft now has a website, Small Business Center and the home page has an article by Kim Komando who gives "4 ways to prevent computer-related injuries." "According to recent numbers from the U. S. Bureau of Labor statistics, more than 100,000 employees missed three to five days of work in the past year to a musculoskeletal disorder." She suggests "The eyes have it, a seat fit for a king, Make your desktop setup functional and user-friendly and Take a break?"

During my research of NIOSH and OSHA, I found an arm of the agency, NORA which is the research portion. In February 2006,

I was invited to present my findings for solving the issue of computer related injuries at Tampa, Fl. and these ideas are being considered regarding left hand usage and prevention of injuries. My final thoughts on exercise before you turn on your computer to work are the same as Elaine Zablocki, who states computer jocks are at risk. If you work at a keyboard for 6 hours or more, go home to play video games and then wonder why your hands feel strange, you are a computer jockey. Any athlete knows you stretch before you work out.

My advice for your consideration is, while your computer is loading the various components, do the routines explained in your book. That is a great way to start your computer work day. Don't forget to remind yourself throughout the day when you take rest breaks a.m. and p.m., stretch your upper body and back too. Have the attitude, I am a Computer Jock or I am a Computer Jill.

# CHAPTER EIGHT

*Silicon Valley is like a person running around in front of a steam-roller. You can outrun the steamroller on any given day. But if you ever sit down you get squashed.*

**Bob Boschert**

## ESTABLISHING DIRECTIONALITY

Your objective in this first training is to assist you in learning how to use the numeric device with the left hand. For some of you this will be your non dominant hand, if you are right handed. For those of you who are left handed or mixed handed, this may or may not be your dominant hand. The inheritance of handedness is vague. Anthony Smith writes in his book, The Body, about Digital Dominance and statistics: 10% of the children of two right handers are left handed but the proportion goes up to 20–25% if the parents are mixed (right and left) and to 30% if both parents are themselves left handed.

## SELECTION OF COMPUTER INPUT DEVICES

The prior special preparation for this training is computer keyboard and keypad training using the right hand side computer and keypad, the regular computer keyboard. If you are at work, following learning the early steps, you may wish to use some of that work for your non- dominant hand work. If your work situation has not provided your numerical keypad device, you may go to www.fentek-ind.com or www.Goldtouch.com, or Kensington on the web and review the types that are available and most suited for your computer and keyboard. I recommend a keypad hub which will allow you to do all your calculations from the keypad. There are 10 key, 17 key and 22 key types of input devices.

When I spoke with Stephen Bucaro in reference to swap buttons or swap keys, he asks the question, but "what if you are left handed?" for the mouse. "One of the biggest benefits of a GUI (Graphical Users Interface) is the fact that you don't need to type everything, many of your tasks can be accomplished by simply clicking on a mouse key. The standard mouse has two buttons, the left button is used to select, open, close, and move element of the interface, and the right button is used to open context menus. About 12 percent of the population is left-handed and they are usually forced to function in a right-handed world. Fortunately, Windows lets you swap the functions of the mouse buttons. It's important to let left-handed people be as productive as possible because, on average, left-handed people are more creative than right-handed people. That's why occupations like designer and architect have a higher percentage of left-handed people than the general population." Mauricio Tejada has a simple version called the DMouse found on the website under computers on anythingleft-handed.com which is free ware.

Design changes occur daily, so check again what key type you need. As of this writing you can find wireless keypads too at www.tigerdirect.com. You also can find a dual keypad at www.piengineering.com. Sierra Rein in her article about programmable keypads at ergnonomicproducts.articleinsider.com writes "a programmable keypad can be instrumental in increasing productivity and enhancing use with any computerized system." This type of "A keypad can reduce typing time and save a lot of effort in the meantime."

## UNDERSTANDING COORDINATION
## OF THE EXTREMITIES

There are important facts you need to know and understand how the anatomy and physiology of your hands, fingers and brain organization allow you to think and do the skills necessary to learn numerical data input. If you have reservations about proceeding with training, I recommend you to go back and review any notes you may have made.

Hand and finger movements have just so many coordinated movements they can make. If you have been typing and completing data entry for a long time with the right hand, this will be old learning. The same is true if you have musical training with a piano, keyboard, violin or guitar, you will have old learning also. Frequently old learning will interfere with new learning. That is the purpose of this training: to help you with the interference within your brain organization and prior learning experiences. It also will be helpful if you understand coordination and how the neurons controlling your arms and nearby leg neurons work together, so they do not disturb each other. Do you recall the simple coordinated movements of patting the top of your head with one hand and with a circular movement with the other hand over your abdominal area? It was usually a side splitter with laughter. Why don't you give that example a try? Well, you will learn more of the importance of that during another coordination experiment.

## CLOCKWISE AND
## COUNTERCLOCKWISE MOVEMENTS

One of the easier coordination tasks is to pat your head with one hand and with the other hand, make a circular motion in front of your abdomen. That is easy. A little more difficult is to make a circular motion with your right arm and try to make a letter 6 (six) with the other arm in space. Now that is difficult.

I first read of this next coordination exercise in the Eric Haseltine article Neuroquest in the Discovery magazine, page 88, March 2002. I have only included parts of the exercise just to show you the importance of how the arms and legs must work together. So, have fun and take this coordination challenge. If you have your family nearby, have them join in too.

You can sit in a chair to do this. Hold out your right arm with your palm down. With your right arm, in a circular motion, like "polishing an imaginary piece of furniture", get a "good rhythm going" and then start your right foot circling in the same direction. That is easy. Now, try the same right arm circling and try to allow your right foot to circle in a counterclockwise direction. Now, that was difficult if not impossible. Dr. Haseltine explains this coordinated effort as "when the neurons controlling your arm and the nearby leg neurons work together, they do not disturb each other much."

The second part of this exercise is, to repeat your right arm circling or polishing motion. But, this time use your left foot. Try the counterclockwise movement. This should be easy because "the control centers for the two limbs inhabit opposite sides of the brain and don't bother each other very much", according to Dr. Haseltine.

Now that you understand coordination, clockwise and counterclockwise movement, you are ready for the use of your handwriting skills. Next we will use this skill test to help us determine the directionality best for you, left to right or right to left. I learned of the importance of directionality from noted psychologist, Theodore Blau, and his development of The Torque Test. It is a test of lateral dominance and over 30 individual research studies have been done using this neuropsychological evaluation test which can be used with children or adults.

The Blau Torque Test is a simple exercise requiring each person to do "use the preferred writing hand and then with the non dominant hand." At your work table with a plain piece of typing paper, draw a line in the middle from the top to the bottom. Then on the right side top, write R-for right. On the left side top, write L-for left. Now, with your right hand and pencil on the right side, draw 3 X's down the page. Then, draw circles around each X. Note which direction, left to right or right to left you make your circles. Repeat the left hand and pencil on the left side, draw 3 X's down the page. Then, draw circles around each X and note which direction, left to right or right to left you make your circles.

If all six of the circlings are all drawn in the same counterclockwise direction, the scoring is no torque. If one or more circlings are done in a clockwise direction, the scoring is torque. There are eight combinations of circling behavior. This test is used with the permission of Dr. L. Blau, Trustee as Dr. Theodore Blau passed away in 2003 in Tampa, Florida. This is the best explanation I have seen for coordination of the hands.

From all of the people and workers who have taken any of the directionality tests, not one person has said it does not matter. I can do it either way. I am reminded of the conversations with a co-worker who not only is a Nurse Case Manager but also left handed.

*Grafton:* Tell me about your experience as your work station was set up for you?

*Kirby:* We live in a world where things are set up to favor right handers. With my first job in computer related worker's compensation medical case management, the IT technician determined since she was left handed, then she should have a left handed clicker on the right side, but she was unable to use the mouse set up for left handers. After a trial of several types of mouse, I was able to use a mouse with the usual clicker on the right side, not the left side.

*Grafton:* So, when you use the numerical keypad on the right, how does that work for you?

*Kirby:* I have no problem with the numbers going left to right.

*Grafton:* What if the keypad was on the left, how would you use that?

*Kirby:* I have to use it the same way, whether it is on the left side or the right side, the numbers have to go left to right. That is the way my brain makes me do it.

Kirby is a parallel learner or shows no torque. So pay close attention to the instructions of the writing test and finger circling test to determine which direction, whether mouse or numerical keypad is most comfortable for you. While reviewing on line at the websites, note the pictures of calculator layouts and the various numerical keyboard and keypad layouts, as you will have decisions to be making as we progress.

## ELIMINATING INTERFERENCE USING THE HANDS AND FINGERS

As an additional exercise we will now use the finger circling task. This one I found in the research. Sit comfortably, you will use both hands. Place your forearms on your work table. Relax your hands. Now take both index fingers, holding the other fingers lightly in. This will be very useful in the second training, Mouse Training. The test is used with the permission of Cortex, a British Journal, from the Wilke-Sheeley study in 1979 at the University of Wisconsin-Parkside and Wright State University entitled Muscular or Directional Preferences in Finger Movement as a Function of Handedness.

"Summary- Right handed, left handed, and "ambiguous" male and female subjects performed circular index finger movements. Analysis of preferred direction of movements showed that strong right handers tend to move both left and right index fingers in the same direction, and familial left handers tend to move them in opposite directions. Since right handers tend to possess a strongly dominant left hemisphere, while familial left handers exhibit a high degree of cerebral lateral equipotentiality, the result indicates that interhemespheric interference in a motor skill consists of activation of inappropriate muscles of the non preferred hand by the dominant ipsilateral (same) hemisphere as its attempts to force that hand to conform to the direction of movement preferred by the dominant hand."

Begin the test with both index fingers pointing but relaxed and comfortable. Make circles with your index fingers. During circumduction (circling), which direction they are moving? Are they both going the same way? If so, that is parallel coordination. If they are going different directions, that is clockwise and counterclockwise or mirror image coordination. By using the results of these tests, this should eliminate any interference you might feel. You may want to review again any pictures of the keypads or mouse from the websites or your own computer keyboard and set up with both directionality patterns to reinforce what you just learned.

Dr. M. K. Holder, a renowned Psychologist at Indiana University with a Research Company has developed an on line questionnaire on handedness that will give an in depth look at handedness and bias in the workplace.

http://www.indiana.edu/~primate/left.html

After completion of his handedness questions, think back in your experiences in sports. Did you ever wonder about switch hitters in baseball? Why some pitchers can throw a screw ball or a curve ball and some cannot? Why some tennis players can serve a slice serve or a kick serve and some cannot? Why some professional golfers swing from the right side for long distance drives but when on the green, putt with their left side? This is dominance in action or your genetic side kicking in allowing the sports player become highly skilled. Now in the case of becoming highly skilled in computer input devices, learn to use your dominance. Again, this is a great genetic dominance family exercise.

## HELP WITH LEARNING

In Perceptual and Motor Skills, (1992) R.A. Rigal in his study of motor control of upper limb and hand, that preference and performance must be used to differentiate the measurement of handedness. Reiss (2000) brings up "hand preference and dexterity between the hands stating handedness is the strongest of motor preferences, descending through footedness and other less known asymmetries (tonguedness, chewing preference)."

All of these tests with no right or wrong answers and exercises should help you feel more comfortable about beginning training your left hand and fingers. You now have determined which directional numerical input device you will begin to use, left to right or right to left. Make sure you are comfortable with which one is comfortable for you.

You may want to use your keypad on your computer or the drawings or notes you may have made using both hands to simulate the use of the keypad. Or your can mentally rehearse by thinking about the whole thing and tapping it out in your mind. Or think about one movement and think about tapping that out in your mind. Or just think about it, period. This is mental rehearsal at its best. Take another look at the keyboards and calculator layouts.

You may be thinking that you are a computer athlete, and that is fine. For skill development you need a mental game showing confidence, focus and determination. You also need a management game which will empower you to look at risk vs. reward, or your skill evaluation. Computer use has become a national past time. Just look at the computer games that people play even after working all day on the computer at work.

If you have had musical training, you may have a metronome already. I strongly support the use of a metronome for the rhythm necessary for data entry input. Also I recommend the use of music with your training sessions. If you are at work, you may wish to use headphones for your music, during your keypad training. I would not start out with fast music but rather work into faster rhythms. Back in the 50s, a musical score of the Typewriter was written, but that is too fast to start with.

Frequently music teachers for piano or guitar will instruct you to do finger exercises. If you are strongly right handed and not participated in the ball sports or musical instruments, I recommend finger exercises daily prior to start of your daily session. The instructions for these were explained earlier. You may want to review those exercises at this time or if you have made notes, review those.

You probably have tried relaxation training before but for a simple explanation, as you sit in your chair, place your hands in your lap, close your eyes, and breathe slowly and deeply. If you have had meditation training, you may want to breathe in from your abdominal muscles and breathe out from your mouth in a slow and rhythmical way. You should try this every day, every hour in your work day. It works wonders. There is always stress at work.

Music often can act as a release from stress. As you respond to music you will have a complex mix of psychological and physiologic reactions according to the article Music Therapy in the Advance for Nurses, Florida Edition, June 27, 2005. Research has shown our heartbeat tends to get in time with music. Music has a calming effect and lessens muscle tension for relaxation. Often interventions are designed to promote wellness, manage stress and enhance memory as well as alleviate pain.

Another trial for easier learning are finger movements on the numerical keypad with your eyes closed, eyes closed and the music beat and also eyes closed and alternating the hands and finger movements. Once you have learned how to perform with your left hand with the keypad input device, I recommend for you to maintain your skill by alternating use of the right and left keypad during the day. Depending upon your job requirement and production required, by alternating you will reduce the keystrokes of your dominant right hand and put some of the overload onto your left hand. This is my explanation of the dual numerical keyboard/keypad set up.

If you are a paid typist, you may be making 9000 keystrokes an hour. If you have had Neurolinguistic Programming training, recall the use of verbs that you use in your communication. Visual learners use see, look, watch, observe etc. Auditory learners use, hear, listen, tell, sounds like. Kinesthetic learners (touch-sensory) use feel, arouse, gut feeling. Also eye access preferences can be noted. Visual learners' eyes will look to the heavens or straight ahead when thinking. Auditory learners may look side to side or look to the non dominant hand. But kinesthetic learners will look to the dominant hand. When you are given instructions in new learning, this is most important to be mindful of, your learning style. When you are prompting yourself with verbal words, try using your favorite words found whether they are visual, auditory and kinesthetic (self talk).

I can recommend reading Bandler and Grindler as their books will help you be more in tune to yourself and others. Richard Restak in his book Mozart and the Fighter Pilot, Restak writes how to enhance your brain power, stating manual and mental skills are not opposed to each other. But they form a continuum. By enhancing your finger and hand motor dexterity, you boost your brainpower.

So practice your chosen manual skill enough to establish and maintain the brain circuits devoted to that skill. By doing this the neurons in your brain will grow microscopic filaments that will connect to one another in the process neuroscientists refer to as arborization. As you master your skills, the brain secretes growth hormones and other chemicals that foster additional arborization. If you fall behind in your practice, the filaments wither away but will not die completely.

During the writing of this book with the training portion, accounting professional Kathy Bakon was interviewed.

*Grafton:* As you reviewed the training exercises with the steps to learning, how did this compare to your numerical training fifteen years ago?

*Bakon:* It was like going back into school again.

## KNOWLEDGE BASE

In both of my computers (GQ Fry's laptop and HP PC), there is the Microsoft XP downloaded system. Check in your computer system by going to Control Panel, click on:

- Click on keyboard
- Click on hardware to customize your keyboard settings.
- In the same control panel look for Mouse.
- Click on Mouse
- Click on hardware to customize your mouse settings. You will probably find the PS2 and the HID listed. The laptop has more types of hardware listed, for example in Mouse settings, left or right. The PC has fewer offerings. In the Control Panel, numerical keypads are not shown. On the PC keyboard, the numerical keypad is standard (generic left to right). On the laptop, the numeric keypad is doubled within the keyboard and can be used with the Fn key and it also is generic, left to right. As more operating systems are improved expect more changes in the Control Panel: Mouse, Keyboard. Many of the new computers are using USB keyboards and mice as opposed to the PS/2 mouse. USB devices are plug and play. You may need to read again the information from Stephen Bucaro and Mauricio Tejada and their swap mouse key solutions for the left hand.

## TYPES OF PC COMPUTER DOMINANCE FOR THE DUAL KEYBOARD METHOD

Due to human factors and brain organization this sequential learning for the non preferred hand will either be parallel sequencing or mirror image sequencing based upon the person's dominance. Following testing of torque in left hand usage for hands and fingers from the Grafton patent, the computer user may have parallel or mirror image directionality as explained by Dr. Theodore Blau in his book published by APA, The Torque Test: A Measurement of Cerebral Dominance, Jan., 1974.

Used with permission of Dr. Theodore Blau Trust by Dr. Lily Blau.

This is an example for you to use as you prepare for purchase of peripheral input devices or an additional keypad for your dual system of keyboarding.

## TESTING RESULTS

NAME _____

COMPANY _____

DATE _____


DOMINANCE (RH, LF, MxH, A)
Right handed, left handed, mixed handed or ambidextrous

_____

HANDWRITING (PARALLEL, MIRROR) FINGER CIRCLING (PARALLEL, MIRROR) _____

_____

DEVICES (PS2, USB, OTHER) _____

_____

KEYPAD _____

CALCULATOR_____

MOUSE OR POINTING DEVICE_____

After completing the various tests for computer dominance for the mouse and keyboard, to set up your Dual Numerical Keyboard Based on Dominance, these are my recommendations based on your results. Find your test results and write in your purchase list for the items.

## A. For the Dual Numerical Keyboard and/or mouse from the patent or the instructions.

- Test Results

1) Right handed for left hand usage for mirror image (both for mouse and keypad)
- Selection
- Numeric Keypad (mirror image)
- Mouse (mirror image) left-handed per Microsoft XP
- Test Results

2) Right handed for left hand usage for parallel image — both for mouse and keypad
- Select
- Numeric Keypad (parallel or standard) — You could just move the keyboard to the left and use your right hand if you do very little keypad work for numbers
- Mouse (standard mouse) — You could just move the mouse around to the left side
- Test Results

3) Right handed for left hand usage for mixed dominance for left hand usage, either one
- Parallel or the other mirror image.
- Select
- Look at 1) and 2) to obtain your direction for mouse or keypad
- Test Results

4) Left handed for left hand usage for mirror image (both for mouse and keypad)
- Select

- Numeric Keypad (mirror image)
- Mouse (mirror image)
- Test Results

5) Left handed for left hand usage for parallel image (both for mouse and keypad)
- Select
- Numeric Keypad (parallel or standard) — You can just move the keyboard to the left and use your left hand if you do very little keypad work for numbers
- Test Results

6) Left handed for left hand usage, for mixed dominance for left hand usage, either one parallel or the other mirror image-both for mouse and keypad.
- Select
- Look at 1) and 2) to obtain your direction for mouse or keypad

**B. Examples from job tasks or medical work restrictions**
- Training Module
- Essentials
- Test Results
- For right handed writing and left hand usage for PC use

7) Write with your right hand and use any from above according to your dominance for left hand usage
- For inability to use the right hand (needs rest) for example
- Training Module
- Transitional Work Program

8) Use any of the above for left hand usage from
- A. according to your dominance for left hand usage
- For inability to use the right hand due to amputation or

trauma or other medical/physical problem
- Keyboarding for Success and Training Modules

9) Use any of the above for left hand usage
- Consider using one-handed typing method

10) Customizing Windows for people with disabilities
- Microsoft offers step-by-step guides using three different Dvorak layouts and the standard QWERTY layouts
- Download layouts from the accessibility page on the Microsoft webpage

**C. Companies or persons wishing to begin a workplace safety program.**
- Keyboarding for Success and Training Modules

**D. Companies wishing to explore computer simulation systems: NASA, DOD.**
- Keyboarding for Success and Training Modules

If you are recovering from a bout of Carpal Tunnel Syndrome, tendonitis or other repetitive strain injury of the right hand and your job requires constant use of the numerical keypad or calculator, it is important to reduce the number of keystrokes with the right hand. The testing result notes you have made should allow you to determine what your needs may be.

Are you ready for some new learning?

# PART FOUR

## TRAINING THE LEFT HAND FOR COMPUTER USAGE

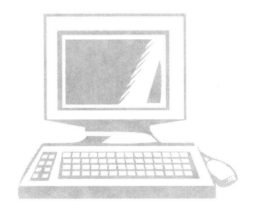

# CHAPTER NINE

*Computers are useless. They can only give you answers.*

**Pablo Picasso**

## DEXTERITY TRAINING
## EDUCATION AND TRAINING

In three weeks of education and training, an hour a day, using this book and your notes, you can significantly improve control of the computer mouse and numerical keypad using your non preferred left hand. Numerical data training has 14 days and mouse training, 7 days.

What is in store for you in the coming chapters are to find out more about your dominance, better understand coordination, pin point your preferences based upon your genetic dominance for input devices and to begin to make logical decisions for changes to your work station. If you wish to learn faster, try a two-a-day session; one in the morning and one in the afternoon.

## THE WILKE-SHEELY STUDY

While researching for the training portion of this book, I found a study that was in agreement with some of my previous research on handedness or laterality. You may need to refer again to the Terms section now. Your curiosity should be up as we move into this information with the training. As you move along, take notes with your questions that will probably find in the closing chapters of the book.

From the web site www.nlm.nih.gov on the subject of laterality, "Book review Laterality, the universe, and everything" the authors discuss genes and their codes. Questions raised are "besides the paraphernalia associated with handedness, the chapters also discuss why clocks go clockwise, why mirrors only appear to reverse right and left,

—Wilke JT, Sheeley EM published in Cortex December 1979

Right handed, left handed, and "ambiguous" male and female subjects performed circular index finger movements. Analysis of preferred direction of movements showed that strong right handers tend to move both left and right index fingers in the same direction, and familial left handers tend to move them in opposite directions. Since right handers tend to possess a strongly dominant left hemisphere, while familial left handers exhibit a high degree of cerebral lateral equipotentiality, the result indicates that interhemispheric interference in a motor skill consists of activation of inappropriate muscles of the non-preferred hand by the dominant ipsilateral hemisphere as its attempts to force that hand to conform to the direction of movement preferred by the dominant hand.

—Used with permission by Dr. Sala at Cortex Publications

and why bath water spirals down the plug-hole in either direction irrespective of whether you are in the Northern or Southern Hemispheres." The authors "suspect the theory will have its greatest impact in governing how we think about asymmetry — especially at the intersections between the disciplines of chemistry, biology, medicine, and psychology."

## A PROGRAMMER'S EXPERIENCE WITH LATERALITY AND PREFERENCES

During the interview with computer programmer expert, Mathew Monroe, we covered his experience using his left hand at work on the computer.

> *Grafton:* Since you had figured out you were mirror image in your brain organization, did you try and use the left hand during numerical data entry?

> *Monroe:* Oh, yes I did try to use the numerical key pad with my left hand. I found it more difficult, because I was mirrored, and the keypad felt backwards to me with my left hand. I did eventually get used to it, but using a left hand right to left numerical keypad was much more effective for me.

Definitely he recommends using a numerical keypad on the left side based on his genetic dominance. In my correspondence with Monroe, his comments are "software and hardware is being geared more toward ambidexterity."

## TRANSFER OF TRAINING BETWEEN THE HANDS

One of the more important studies is the Wilke and Sheeley study of muscular or directional preferences in finger movement as a function of handedness concluded in their "analysis of preferred direction of movements showed that strong right handers tend to move both left and right index fingers in the same direction, and familial left handers tend to move them in opposite directions." Their results indicated that "interhemispheric interference in a motor skill consists of activation of inappropriate muscles of the non preferred hand by the dominant ipsilateral (same) hemisphere as its attempts to force that hand to conform to the direction of movement preferred by the dominant hand."

Now that we have a better understanding of how the hands work together easily then we look at experiments to see if there is help for either hand as you learn to become more dexterous. We know from the Jancke study (2000) that through "use of the MRI, signals change in the sensorimotor cortex to finger movements of a different rate of the dominant hand and the sub dominant hand."

Several studies answer the question if your dominant right hand will influence your training of the left hand. These findings suggest that a task already learned by one hand can positively influence the learning of the same task by the other hand. The results have important implications for occupational therapy — namely, that activities comprising tasks previously learned by one hand would be more effective in facilitating improved performance by the other hand than activities comprising previously unlearned tasks in the case of retraining skills in patients with amputation or hemiplegia. From these studies, you can see the importance of applying this book of training the left hand for our veterans who may have lost the use of the right hand from trauma or amputation.

Once you have completed the handwriting test and the finger circling test, you will begin to understand and conclude, yes I have dominance. And, now I know what my genetic dominance is between my hands and my hand and finger to finger and their preferred direction as far as using a numerical device or mouse with my left hand. Now I know what to do with my genetic dominance.

Don't let that confuse you? Just look at both of your hands, then slightly flex your index fingers. On your table or computer, tap out with your fingers with the numbers which one feels best for you, left to right or right to left. This should be the same as your test results for the left hand, parallel or mirror image coordination.

Following this numerical keypad training, you may wish to establish a dual system of keypads as this will allow you to rest your right hand and fingers if you job requires mostly numeric data entry with a small amount of keyboard work.

What is new on the market is the "Human Interface Hardware" designed by PI Engineering on their website. You will find a high resolution picture of the X-keys Desktop Programmable Keypad. The X-keys come with a precut sheet of legends which can easily be written on or run through a printer. Clear caps cover the legends to keep them from wearing off. For the purposes of the numbers pad, I would recommend the PS/2 version of the X-keys. It is incredibly easy to program and comes with two double-tall keys and one double-wide key so that it may easily be configured to mimic the numbers pad for either hand. The other version they offer, the USB version, is best for laptops, (when you aren't using a full sized keyboard, and systems that do not have a PS/2 keyboard port (Apple). Regarding the numbers pad, the X-keys Desktop (http://www.piengineering.com/xkeys/xkdesk.php) would be perfect for this. The X-keys supports two layers of programming, so it would be a simple matter of programming the numbers in one direction on the green layer and the opposite direction on the red layer and using a layer toggle key to switch between them. Also the numbered key caps (part # XK-A-246) can be purchased by going to their website.

Globlink's breakthrough design combines the functions of wireless numerical keypad and trackball mouse, available for both left and right-handed users. Globlink also makes a wireless keyboard with an optical trackball with a mouse that has left and right keys.

In the "History of Personal Workstations" by Dr. A. Goldberg in 1988, she explained "It is clear that all of the most important innovations in Human-Computer Interaction (HCI) have benefited from research at both corporate research labs and universities, much of it funded by the government. The conventional style of graphical user interfaces that use windows, icons, menus and a mouse and are in a phase of standardization, where almost everyone is using the same, standard technology and just making minute, incremental changes." In another discussion Dr. Golberg states "Another important argument in favor of HCI research in universities is that computer science students need to know about user interface issues. User interfaces are likely to be one of the main value-added competitive advantages of the future, as both hardware and basic software become commodities. If students do not know about user interfaces, they will not serve industry needs." (That is why my system of dual keyboarding is so important.) "As computers get faster, more of the processing power is being devoted to the user interface. The interfaces of the future will use gesture recognition, speech recognition and generation, 'intelligent agents' to name a few." If the computer user is to keep up with innovations in speed of new products, it will behoove you to look at dexterity training seriously. One question you may have is; will dexterity training change my life as I change my workstation? My best answer is through increased networking between the two halves of the brain you will become more skilled with the use of your hands and fingers. You will need to make choices to stay in the computer game.

Is the electronic industry the only one interested in longevity and productivity? The sports industry for years has been involved with studies regarding left handers and right handers. In a syndicated article "Switch pitcher debuts" in New York, June 2008, between the Staten Island Yankees and the Brooklyn Cyclones made his debut and confounded the umpires as the switch handed batter coming to the plate kept changing sides and the pitcher changed with each of the batter's moves. The umpire was perplexed. After meeting with the opposing coaches and the umpires it was concluded by ruling the batter must make a choice before coming to the plate and the pitcher will accommodate.

Baseball is not the only game with switch hitting. In the case of the tennis professional coach at Syracuse University and ESPN announcer, Luke Jensen, confounding the opposition with skillful serving with both the left hand and the right hand in tennis matches was the norm during the 80s. In tennis, the server makes the choice prior to serving each serve, first serve or second serve. Generally, the right handed server has an advantage in the right court and the left handed server has the advantage of serving in the left court.

You have a choice. You may be externally motivated for change from a helping or a learning objective (hand pain) or a self drive or internal motivation objective (life success/productivity) with use of your hands and fingers at your computer workstation. The dual numerical keyboard/keypad and/or mouse are the concepts of saving your hands and increasing your productivity and longevity by re distribution of your job tasks with dexterity training.

# CHAPTER TEN

*One of the most feared expressions in modern times is "The computer is down."*

**Norman Augustine**

## NUMERICAL DATA TRAINING (KEYPAD)

Daily steps (14) for learning numerical or calculator data entry with the left hand

## LESSONS IN STEPS

Each step is a lesson for the day. You may want to purchase a yellow pad for your daily work log. Allow an hour for each lesson.

### The First Day

*Step 1*

- Position Check: Your computer keyboard/keypad in place. Assemble your left numerical input device in place to the left of your keyboard/keypad. Are your feet flat on the floor?

*Step 2*

- Is your keyboard/keypad or keypads in front of you? Make sure you have enough room. Is your computer monitor squarely in front of you? Is it high enough so you can maintain your posture? I have included in this chapter a checklist, so you will see the importance of your workstation and your posture.

## Step 3

- Did you decide your left to right or right to left directionality for your numerical keypad? I have given instructions for the mirror image directionality. If you are a parallel type, then do the same as you would with the right side keypad with left to right direction.

## Step 4

- With all new learning there is stress, so take some slow deep breaths (diaphragmatic breathing).
- Now dangle your arms down at your sides. Now take your left hand and place your index finger on 4, middle finger on 5 and 4th finger on 6. Press 4, then 5, then 6, then Enter.
- Do this 3 times.

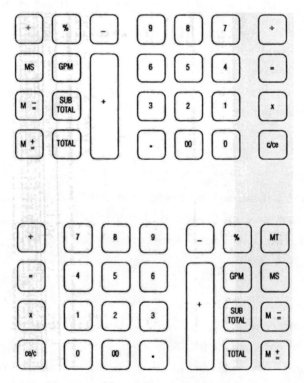

*Numerical keypads numbers locations.*

- Your screen should show:

  456

  456

  456

- Now practice this: After pressing the number 3 times then press Enter.

  444 555 666 456, do this 3 times

  456 654 456 654, do this 3 times

## Step 5

- Learn the 1, 2, 3, keys
- Now press 1 with your index finger, 2 with your middle finger and 3 with your 4th finger.
- After each finger press, return to the basic finger position of 4, 5 and 6. Do this 3 times.

  123 123 123 123 123 123 123 123 123

- Now practice this: Press Enter after 3 numbers.

  414 141 411 144 441 414

  525 252 522 255 552 225

  636 336 663 366 363 636

## Step 6

- Learn the 7, 8, 9 keys
- Your fingers should be in your basic position. Press 7 with your index finger, 8 with your middle finger and 9 with your 4th finger. After each finger press, return to the basic finger position of 4, 5 and 6. While your fingers are in the basic position, with your little finger, press Enter. Do this 3 times.

  777 888 999

  777 888 999

  474 475 744 766 746 547

  696 969 669 996 474 547

  855 855 844 854 856 658

## Step 7

- While your fingers are in the basic position, with your little finger, press +, then Enter after 3 presses. Do this 3 times

+++ +++ +++ +++ +++ +++

## Step 8

- While your fingers are in the basic position, with your little finger, press -. Do this 3 times.

— - — - — - — - — - — —

## Step 9

- With your fingers in the basic position, with your index finger, go up 2 places and press Num Lock, then with your middle finger go up 2 places and press /, then with your 4th finger go up 2 places and press *. After each finger press, return to the basic finger position of 4, 5 and 6.

## Step 10

- Depending upon your keyboard, keypad device, you may not need your left thumb exercise portion, if not please pass this next paragraph.

## Step 11

- With your fingers in the basic position, press with your thumb each directional arrow, return each time to the basic position. You should be more comfortable now, just knowing where the numbers are. Now can you do the entire exercise without looking?

## Step 12

- Learn the 0 and decimal keys
- Use the thumb for the 0 and the third finger for the (.)
- Now practice this, pressing Enter to accomplish this task.

3.5 3.8 6.9 .5 .6 .7 5.64 6.45

4056 802 .30 3.06 6045 2.8

- This is your basic drill.

## The Second Day
### Step 1
- Repeat the basic drill.

### Step 2
- This next step will help you focus on performance, speed and accuracy. For this step you will need a watch or clock. Keep a log book on how long it takes you to complete the basic drill.

### Step 3
- Review each day your progress. Use date, goal is speed, goal is accuracy, errors, time spent, other notations.

## The Third Day
### Step 1
- Repeat the basic drill.

### Step 2
- During this step, increase your total numbers input from 3 numbers to 6 numbers. For example, 1, 2, 3, 4, 5, 6, 3 times.

### Step 3
- Then 4, 5, 6, 7, 8, 9, 3 times. Do not look at the keys, focus on the numbers. If you are using your metronome, complete the drill again, focus on rhythm. Are you able to complete the drill with the use of music? If you feel a 'brain block' at any time, you can close your eyes and go through the numbers without looking. You can also use finger movements with the eyes closed to music. And you can also use closing your eyes

and alternating your hands for your finger movements. Record your progress.

## The Fourth Day
### *Step 1*
• Repeat the basic drill.

### *Step 2*
• The secret of performance is concentration and keeping your mind on each number. You may find at this time it will help you to say each number before you press that number.

### *Step 3*
• So, repeat Lesson 1, 2, and 3 and verbalize each step. Determine if verbalizing helps or hinders your performance. Record your progress.

## The Fifth Day
### *Step 1*
• Repeat the basic drill.
• Has this become a habit, reviewing each lesson with the steps?

### *Step 2*
• Learning good technique in use of the computer and keypad requires emphasis on speed.
• How much time does it take to complete the basic drill?

### *Step 3*
• This motor skill needs to be developed through the steps and exercises. If you will focus on speed and rhythm, your accuracy will follow. Spend your time this session on speed and rhythm. Record your progress.

**The Sixth Day**
*Step 1*
- Repeat the basic drill. Note how you are improving.

*Step 2*
- Repeat Lesson 2 and 3
- Accuracy is also required in keypad data entry. Spend your time this session on accuracy.

*Step 3*
- Record your progress. Which steps show greater improvement?

**The Seventh Day**
*Step 1*
- You should be comfortable knowing where the keypad numbers are with your left hand.
- Review again the basic drill.

*Step 2*
- This session, alternate the exercises first with the right hand. Then, the same exercises with the left hand. Key stroke as fast as you can.

*Step 3*
- Did you verbalize? How was your rhythm on each side? Is your data entry from your right hand essentially the same as your left hand? Do you still look at the left hand while keying?

*Step 4*
- If you do, repeat some of the steps with the left hand before you move to the next step.

**The Eighth Day**
*Step 1*
• Repeat the basic drill then repeat Lesson 4 and 5

*Step 2*
• In this step, get accustomed to typing and keying which is a part of billing, letter writing and other types of office work. This may be a part of your job, so finding the work will be easy. But, if you are at home, look at your own bill paying system work and separate out some of the paper work to include with your session today.

**The Ninth Day**
*Step 1*
• Repeat the basic drill. Repeat Lesson 7 and 8

*Step 2*
• After you have practiced your basic steps, now complete the numbers 1, 2, 3, 4, 5, 6, 7, 8, 9, 0 —3 times.

*Step 3*
• You should feel comfortable knowing where the numbers are with the left hand.

*Step 4*
• Now alternate to the right hand, the same exercise, — 1 time.

*Step 5*
• Alternate 3 times left hand, then right hand.

*Step 6*
• Is your data entry from right hand to left hand rhythmic? Is speed difficult? Are errors numerous? Does verbalizing the

numbers help?

### Step 7
• Complete the exercise again, alternating hands, right and left. Record your progress.

## The Tenth Day
### Step 1
• Repeat the basic drill. Repeat Lesson 9

### Step 2
• In his session, concentrate on improvement of your motor skill of the left hand. To increase your speed of the left hand data entry, practice, practice, practice. As you begin your session, have a goal in mind. Will it be speed today or accuracy today?

### Step 3
• You can only concentrate on one thing at a time. Select your goal for the session. Pick out at least 2 exercises.

### Step 4
• Is verbalizing helping? If so, then do that. Record your progress.

## The Eleventh Day
### Step 1
• Repeat the basic drill and Lesson 10

### Step 2
• Data keying and typing are skills that must be exercised. You will need self discipline to accomplish your goal of using the non dominant hand for numerical data entry with speed and accuracy. Set a goal everyday. That goal may be, complete the

step without interruption.

## Step 3

- Complete the step with less than 3 errors. If you are having difficulty with verbalizing, set a goal aloud before keying so that you can control your fingers.

## Step 4

- When working on your speed goal, push yourself. Keep a daily practice record of your progress. Review your speed and accuracy. Know you will have good days and bad days, but you will improve with your goal setting. Record you progress today and set your goals for the next session.

## Step 5

- Review your log. Have you made notes as to what is working well for you and what is not?

## The Twelfth Day
### Step 1

- Repeat the basic drill and then, review your personal lessons learned in Lesson 11.

## Step 2

- Do you remember your adding skills learned at school? $1 + 1 = 2, 2 + 2 = 4, 3 + 3 = 6, 4 + 4 = 8,$
- $5 + 5 = 10, 6 + 6 = 12, 7 + 7 = 14, 8 + 8 = 16, 9 + 9 = 10.$ Do this exercise 3 times.

## Step 3

- Alternate with the right hand, 1 time.

*Step 4*
- Complete the exercise again with the left hand, 3 times.

*Step 5*
- Complete the exercise with speed in mind, 1 time.

*Step 6*
- Complete the exercise with accuracy in mind, 1 time. Record your progress.

## The Thirteenth Day
*Step 1*
- Repeat your basic drill. Review and repeat Lesson 12.

*Step 2*
- Persevere. Learning to use the left hand can be fun and it can also be rewarding. If you work for a bank, you will probably be paid a basic salary plus production. By resting your right hand and using the left hand frequently, you will become more powerful in the use of your hands and all the while increasing your brains neurons. If you work in Human Resources, that type of office puts greater stress on accuracy than on speed. If you are going to take an employment test, you may remind the tester, you are able to use both hands now on numerical data entry, if that is part of the test.

*Step 3*
- You have learned how to relax just by putting your arms down and breathing deeply, slowly several times.

*Step 4*
- Now for today's session. Data entry today is organization based using tens and units.

- For example 45 + 5= 50, now 40 + 5+ 5 = 50, now 30 + 5 + 5 + 5 + 5 = 50. That is easy, correct? Now let us try patterns and order. 8, 16, 24, 32, 40, 48, 56, 64, 72, 80, 88, 96, 104, 112, 120, 128. Calculate the total.

### Step 5

- Now 9, 18, 27, 36, 45, 54, 63, 72, 81, 90, 99, 108. Calculate the total.

### Step 6

- The second part of this session is patterns with numbers. $9 \times 9 + 7 =$ calculate, $98 \times 9 + 6 =$ calculate, $987 \times 9 + 5 =$ calculate, $9876 \times 9 + 4 =$ calculate, $98765 \times 9 = 3 =$ calculate, $987654 \times 9 + 2 =$ calculate, $9876543 \times 9 + 1 =$ calculate.

### Step 7

- Now let us try simple totals. Please add these dollar amounts 122.50, 200.00, 400.00, 300.00, 50.00, 50.00. Calculate total.

### Step 8

The second trial.

- 30,873.00, 96,000.00, calculate. Record your progress.

### The Fourteenth Day
### Step 1

- Repeat the basic drill. Repeat Lesson 13 with all of the calculations.

### Step 2

- You should be very familiar with the keypad numbers on the left side and more than familiar with those on the right side. This next drill will use amounts and credits with the balance similar to the facts from banking and finance.

- Key in 10.00 + 19.98 + 12.71 + credit 1,035.79 + 16.03 + 59.96 + 34.98 + 39.56 + 18.00 + 21.51. Calculate the total.

## Step 3
- Do this 2 times with the left keypad, then 1 time with the right hand.

## Step 4
- Then compare the time it took for the left hand calculation and the right hand calculation.

## Step 5
- Were they close in timing? If not, then you may wish to look at one your statements from your credit card account or your bank account and give them a try on each side, time them and compare. Or if you are at work, compare some of your work with the left hand keypad work with your right hand keypad work. Record your progress.

## Step 6
- In the next chapters, I will bring to your attention some of your questions you probably have. For example, what about touch? Performance? Why do some people learn faster than others, especially motor (muscle) skills? With all of this information what more should I know? Keep your mind open to what more that you just may be interested in. You have just completed the basic 14 lessons with steps to provide you with Ambidexterity Training for the numerical keypad or calculator.

# CHAPTER ELEVEN

*The pain of not doing something is greater than the pain of doing something.*

**William Dennis Miner**

## FINDING YOUR TARGET

As you begin your personal journey to reconfigure your computer workstation, consider what your job requirements are and the skills needed to increase your productivity or just simply for your convenience. You also may wish to take a look at the description of the job you are in.

Let us review your test results on handedness first. Most of us are strong right handers or dextrals. Also most of us use the standard mouse with the left clicker for the right index finger and the middle finger (3rd) for point and drag. Most of us also use our right hand for handwriting. Even computer users who have taken this training, say they began using the mouse on the left side "just for convenience" for them. You can increase your productivity just by moving your mouse to the left hand side using your left hand and continue your writing tasks with your right hand. That will save time by not having to take the time to look for your pen or pencil and then look for your mouse.

## DEFINING YOUR HAND AND FINGER PREFERENCES FOR THE MOUSE

If you choose not to purchase a programmable mouse or a left handed mouse, then simply move your mouse to the left hand side, substitute your 3rd finger for your index finger and your index finger for your 3rd finger. After you learn how to use your left hand for the mouse and you wish to use a dual mouse system (one for each hand), P. I. Engineering makes a Y mouse adapter which provides a fast, easy means to connect to two mice to a single port. The price from the web site $49.95. You can check the website www.ymouse.com and view other input devices. From the programmers and CAD Operators standpoint, you may need this right away.

Hoffman E. and Chang (1997) at the University of Melbourne in Australia, surveyed student-use computers and found that "100% had the mouse installed on the right-hand side." In their experiment to "determine if the left-handed user was disadvantaged" by this arrangement, the findings, as expected, "left-handers were found to be superior to right-handed users when using their non-preferred left hand" (245–8).

You may have noticed that a mouse can be mice when you are talking about more than one mouse. Too, the mouse is often called a pointing device. If you will recall, the index finger is referred to as the pointer finger.

Keir P., Bach and Rempel (1999) at the University of California in San Francisco studied the effects of computer mouse design and task on carpal tunnel pressure. Just as "computer mouse use has become an integral part of office work, intensive mouse use has been associated with RSI, MSD and CTS." In this study, "participants performed a multidirectional dragging (drag and drop) task. Recommendations made following the study of 14 healthy subjects are to 1)minimize wrist extension, 2) minimize prolonged dragging tasks, and 3) perform other tasks with the mousing hand" (245–8).

Delisle A., Imbleau, Santos, Planondon, Montpetit (2004) at the

Occupational Health and Safety Research Institute in Quebec, Canada studied "documentation of the impact of using the mouse on the left side of a standard keyboard (with a right numeric keypad) on upper-extremity posture. After one month of ergonomics training shoulder flexion and abduction, as well as wrist extension were reduced with left-handed mouse use." For work involving both keyboard and mouse use, and without the need of the numeric keypad it would probably be preferable to use a keyboard without the numeric keypad if the mouse is to be used on the right-hand side. A final comment of the study "an interesting alternative would be to use the mouse on the left side provided sufficient time is allowed to get accustomed to it."

Are you getting ready to take the time to save you time?

Globlink Technology, Inc. has developed a revolutionary technology transforming your Eyeshot. A tiny, compact size and easily transported for the laptop is a USB type of mouse with a left key and right key with a scroll wheel. Globlink also makes a wireless keyboard with an optical trackball with a mouse that has left and right keys. This company has also developed a Ring Mouse and Bracelet Mouse. In an article on WebMD by Jennifer Warner, she states Typing Rarely Cause of Carpal Tunnel, but "your mouse could be a little worse than working on a keyboard", from the article June 10, 2003. Don't forget to review websites for swap keys or swap buttons. They give all of the instructions starting with Control Panel, then Mouse.

## HOME OFFICE WORKER INTERVIEW

Another story of a home office worker who deals in real estate and financial investing gave this account of his workstation.

*Grafton:* What is the reason you have a left handed mouse on the right side of the computer, especially since you are right handed?

*Dennis D.:* The reason I have the back handed click is, I use a track ball with the right hand, manipulating the ball with my index and middle finger and clicking with my ring finger. I find this very easy. Back clicking (the left button) takes a little extra motion with my index finger. Holding down the right button with the ring finger while moving the ball with my middle and index finger is much easier to coordinate than using my index finger to hold down the left button and moving the ball with the middle finger.

*Grafton:* How did you get started with that set up?

*Dennis D.:* I ended up this way because I used to work with a lefty who always reversed the buttons on the track balls because he was the 'computer guy'. I got used to it. But, it seems that the 'righty' set up was better for the mouse than for track balls.

Peters M., and Ivanoff (1999) at the Dept. of Psychology in Guelph, Ontario, Canada studied performance by right-handers and left-handers with right-handed mouse experience and by left-handers with left-handed mouse experience. They "recorded measures of reaction time, time to reach a target, time to click on target and cursor trajectory. Precision and general directional aiming with the mouse cursor showed clear right hand superiority in the mouse users on the right side." But, they determined "the difference could be reduced with practice." When there is a need to forestall or ameliorate repetitive stress in the experienced right hand, then consider left hand mouse use training.

**MAKING YOUR DECISION**

At this time of reconciling yourself to change, consider continuing to write with your right hand and move or buy the non standard mouse for use on the left hand side with the clicker for your left hand index finger on the right side of the mouse. Did you decide on the standard or non standard mouse? Check your result list and adjust your keyboard if needed. Did you decide if you are right handed? Or, left handed? Or a mixed hander? Did you need to check your job description if it says anything about use of the hands at your work station? Sometimes the phrase "must use right hand by touch" for tools in the work place. Will it help you to move your mouse to the left hand side of the computer? If you believe it will help in your job performance or with any medical problems at your work station, consider it a trial or a must see if will help.

Will it help to use two hands learning mouse training? Generally using two hands for skills are for lack of strength, i.e. two handed backhand in tennis. If you are disabled with the right hand but still have your extremity, you could certainly give it a try. But, you may generate more interference within yourself which could impede your performance. If you job requires excessive mouse use, then you may wish to consider a dual handed mouse set up. Computer programmers often have dual mouse set ups. If you are having trouble with the index finger (your pointer finger) on your right hand, you may wish to consider this training for sure.

Remember, intensive use of the computer keyboard, keypad and mouse increases the risk of development of work-related musculo-skeletal symptoms in the shoulders too, right along with your upper and lower arms, wrists, hands and fingers. So, spread your tasks among both sides of your computer work station. This includes your writing hand, telephone or any other device that you use frequently. All of these steps will help you with your job productivity plus saving your hands.

Before we begin, check out the instructions on your mouse again. Was it programmable? Wireless? Are you a mirrored individual or a parallel individual in your brain organization? Make sure you are comfortable with all of those decisions. So, let us work on target training using the left hand for your mouse pointing movements.

As you begin your personal journey to reconfigure your computer workstation, consider what your job requirements are and the skills needed to increase your productivity. Let us review your test results on handedness first. Most of us are strong right handers or dextrals. Also most of us use the standard mouse with the left clicker for the right hand. But, we also use our right hand for handwriting. You can increase your productivity just by moving your mouse to the left hand side using your left hand and continue your writing tasks with your right hand.

## RESEARCH ABOUT THE MOUSE

You may have noticed that a mouse can be mice when you are talking about more than one mouse. Too, the mouse is often called a pointing device. At this time of reconciling yourself to change, consider continuing to write with your right hand and move or buy the non standard mouse for use on the left hand side with the clicker for your left hand index finger on the right side of the mouse. Did you decide on the standard or non standard mouse? Check your result list and adjust your keyboard if needed. Did you decide if you are right handed? Or, left handed? Or a mixed hander?

Did you need to check your job description if it says anything about use of the hands at your workstation? Sometimes the phrase "must use right hand by touch" for tools in the work place. Will it help you to move your mouse to the left hand side of the computer? If you believe it will help in your job performance or with any medical problems at your work station, consider it a trial or a must see if will help.

In other research of the use of the fingers (digits), a Biological Scientist Dr. Ranganathan (2001) studied skilled finger movement and concluded exercise improves hand function, so it is worthwhile to continue your hand and finger exercises to keep up with modernization. Dr. Kornatz and his partners in Applied Physiology in

2005 concluded practice reduces motor unit discharge variability in a hand muscle and improves manual dexterity.

Before we begin, check out the instructions on your mouse again. Was it programmable? Wireless? Are you a mirrored individual or a parallel individual in your brain organization? Make sure you are comfortable with all of those decisions. So, let us work on training the left hand for your mouse pointing movements.

Remember, the mind is like a parachute, it works best when it is opened.

# CHAPTER TWELVE

*Do not quench your inspiration and your imagination.*
**Vincent van Gogh**

## MOUSE TRAINING

Each step is a lesson for the day. Have your daily log book yellow pad out too. Allow an hour for each day's lesson. This is important training. From the National Library of Medicine website, when I typed in the search screen, computers, mouse training, there were 514 studies to review.

## LESSONS IN STEPS
### The First Day
### *Step 1*
- Check your test results and determine if you need to use a standard or non standard mouse for the left hand side of the keyboard. Check to see if the mouse is working. You may need to move your computer keyboard slightly to your right giving you more space on the left side for the training. From computer mouse studies women have shorter arms than men. This includes shoulders not as wide. Take into account for this as you become comfortable at your work station.

### Step 2

- You may wish to refer again to the various checklist results you made before you proceed. Again, check the results of whether your directionality is parallel or mirrored as this has importance during the pointing maneuvers.

### Step 3

- With all new learning there is stress, so take some slow deep breaths. You learned earlier this is called diaphragmatic breathing. Dangle your arms down at your sides. Without looking, place your left hand on the mouse. With your dominance and directionality noted, if you are mirrored and using your left index finger on the right side clicker, ok, click it. Then with your 3rd finger or middle finger, ok, just click it. If you are parallel, just place the mouse on the left hand side and proceed. Your 3rd finger will be your pointer and your index finger used for drag and drop. Alternate clicking with the left hand mouse, index finger 3 times. Then the middle finger 3 times.
- This is your basic drill using the mouse on the left hand side.

### The Second Day
### Step 1

- Repeat the basic drill

### Step 2

- Pull up a blank Word or Works document on your computer screen. Save As, Mouse Training.
- Place a bold x on the left side, middle, right side on at least 3 or 4 lines. Use at least 5 lines separating each line of xs.

### Step 3

- In your finger circling result, did you start over or under? This is important, as you want to start either at the top (over) or the bottom (under) of your lines. If you are mirrored start you're pointing to the right side of the screen moving right to left. But, if you are parallel, start at the left side of the screen for your task assignment moving left to right.

### Step 4

- Now that you know your best directionality moves, then with your mouse and finger task, point to each of these xs, without moving the xs. Practice moving to the targets with precision. Do this 3 times.

### Step 5

- Save this document, you will use it again. Save it as Mouse Training if you have not already done so.

## The Third Day

### Step 1

- Review basic drill from Lesson 1

### Step 2

- Pull up your Mouse Training document

### Step 3

- Review your finger pointing task from Lesson 2. Complete the same tasks.

### Step 4

- With your cursor drag each of the xs to the opposite side of the document, and then move them back again. For the middle x, move it to the right or left side and move the x back again

### Step 5

- Record your progress and make any notes for reminders.

## The Fourth Day
### Step 1
- Review basic drills. Look through some of your Saved Documents.

### Step 2
- In your Word documents, pull up one that has text. In the file menu, save as Mouse.
- Click and move some of the sentences, but do not Delete. Now we are going to start the drag and drop task.

### Step 3
- Move each paragraph either above or below the next paragraph. Become accustomed to these tasks and this new learning will soon become old learning. From prior learning, performance comes with practice, practice and more practice. Continue moving your paragraphs for 5 more minutes. Then move them back to where they were at the start of the lesson.

## The Fifth Day
### Step 1
- Pull up your Word document Mouse Training. Point and drag and drop the x's in various up and down positions on your page. This is a warm up drill. Move them back to the prior start of the page. Do this 3 times.

### Step 2
- Pull up your Word document Mouse. Move the cursor to the File menu, click and review, and then back to the page. Move the cursor to the Edit menu, click, review, and then back to the page. Do this with each of the menus, View, Insert, Format, Tools, Table, window or any other at the tables, each time moving back to your page.

*Step 3*

- Pick out in your personal to do list on the computer, do some of your usual work but use your cursor practiced with your training using documentation in Word or Works.

**The Sixth Day**

*Step 1*

- Pull up in Word, one of your documents and use Save as Practice. You can use the following to move through Word, keystrokes, vertical/horizontal scroll bars or Go To to Replace.
- Move through each of these in your document 3 times.

*Step 2*

- Pull up the same document at the start of this lesson. Pull up View. Make a selection and move text at random, 3 times.

*Step 3*

- Pull up the same document again. This time launch Reading Layout. You can increase or decrease text size by + or -. Do this 3 times.

*Step 4*

- Pull up the same document again. You can use the Document Map by choosing View, then Document Map, click a heading and go to that section of the document. Do this 3 times.

*Step 5*

- Again, pull up the same document. Use the Tools menu, Auto Summarize. Look through each of the Windows and view what is shown. Repeat 3 times.

**The Seventh Day**
*Step 1*
- Pull up your Practice document. You can set the Zoom Level by pulling down the View menu, clicking Zoom. Change the Zoom level 3 times.

*Step 2*
- Use the same Practice document. This time, change the Font size. You can apply a new font/type size using the toolbar route by making sure the Formatting toolbar is visible. Select the text you want to amend by using the drop down list, type in the type size you need and press Enter. Do this 3 times.

*Step 3*
- Check out all the menus in your Word or Works program and challenge yourself to moving quickly and confidently with the use of your mouse with the left hand.

*Step 4*
- In your Office program, if you have Excel, PowerPoint, Access, move within those programs to the menus becoming familiar with all of the programs you use frequently.

*Step 5*
- Check your log sheet. Did you make any points that will help increase your performance? Check your log sheet for any of your notes.

*Step 6*
- This concludes your mouse training. Now that you are trained for mouse training with the left hand, congratulate yourself for a job well done. Remember why you chose to take a critical look at your work station. Also remember why you decided to

make a change in your work direction. Intensive use of the computer keyboard, keypad and mouse increases the risk of development of work-related musculoskeletal symptoms in the shoulders too, right along with your upper and lower arms, wrists, hands and fingers. So, spread your tasks among both sides of your computer work station. This includes your writing hand, telephone or any other device that you use frequently.

# PART FIVE

## ENDLESS POSSIBILITIES

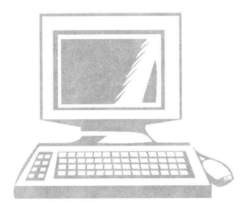

# CHAPTER THIRTEEN

*The real danger is not that computers will begin to think like men, but that men will begin to think like computers.*

**Sidney J. Harris**

## BRAIN ORGANIZATION AND NETWORKING

Surely you have written notes to ask why, or why that or why not this or that? Information in how our brain is organized should help with those questions. Artificial Intelligence (AI) addressed the continuous network of billions of neurons connected to neural nets. These nets explain the mind is not all in the brain but reach out to the sensory organs, such as the eyes and ears. The perceiving human mind of touch, hearing, seeing, tasting and smelling was the basis for the development of machine intelligence. You have noticed my comparisons of the human brain and the computer. Who writes the software programs? The cerebral cortex does. After practice, then the basal ganglia take over the programs. What part of the brain establishes networks? The association cortex does. There are over 100 or so billion neurons that can potentially communicate with any other via one or more of the linkages in the networks according to Dr. Richard Restak.

## CONNECTIONS BETWEEN THE
## BRAIN AND THE HANDS

There appears to be an overlap of control between the two halves of the brain according to the book The Human Body and How it Works. The author explains the "left hemisphere, exercises normal control of the right hand, but less than full control over the left hand; similarly with the right hemisphere." The "right hemisphere is much more successful in recognizing patterns" in movements. In the Science Journal in 1993, S. G. Kim writes in his book about the whole brain and the half brain, there are bundles of 200 million nerve fibers that connect the two halves or hemispheres of the human brain. It is no wonder no two brains are alike in any respect.

In an interview with Danick, Computer Consultant, we brainstormed about "The human brain and networking."

*Grafton:* How can you compare the computer with hardware and software to the human brain (part of the body)?

*Danick:* It depends on what you mean by *Networking?* If you are a talking about it in terms of messages and data moving around, back-and-forth pathways in the mind, comparing them to individual computers and how data moves inside them, that's one discussion, or if you talk about how data moves through the human mind and comparing that to networks built on either Ethernet wire or WiFi Wireless, that's another networking comparison. If you are talk about memory, and being able to recall information that you haven't accessed in years, there's another form of mind and technology networks to discuss. If you talk about recall, the ability to remember and access memories from a taste, a smell, any concept peripherally related to an experience, there's another technology and networking description that an apply.

If you are new at computers you may not understand the complexities he mentions. But if you are a computer programmer, you know for sure what he is talking about. Brain organization and handedness with preference has been researched at great length by numerous professional researchers, (Psychology, Neuroscience, Radiology, Brain, Neurology, and Motor Learning). Although functional lateralization in the human brain has been studied intensively, there continues controversy over the brain mechanisms. What does handedness or use of your hands and fingers have to do with brain lateralization? Review the picture of the brain and hands. Understand?

## EARLY BELIEFS OF THE BRAIN AND MIND

Human handedness and scalp hair-whorl direction develop from a common genetic mechanism according to this study by A. J. Klar in Genetics in 2003. The causes of right-or left-hand preference in human vary from a purely learned behavior, to solely genetics, to a combination of the two mechanisms is Klar's explanation. Did you know that several hundred years ago dominance was selected by your hair whorl? Just by looking at the top of the child's head, noting what direction the hair was growing was the method used. The double hair whorl was a sign of ambidexterity. Klar's statement about the general public consists mostly of right-handers shows clockwise but counterclockwise whorl rotation infrequently (8.4% of individuals). He concludes non-right-handers display a random mixture of clockwise and counterclockwise swirling patterns.

Researchers agree there are undoubtedly differences in cerebral lateralization and other features of brain organization which correlate with hand preference and proficiency as a trait variable according to Wilkes and Sheely. They propose left handers are a heterogenous group, some having a dominant right hemisphere and others having a dominant left hemisphere. These varying patterns of brain hardware, in interaction with environmental experience in a dominantly right handed culture, are likely to produce differences in the fine structure of movement organization.

The Department of Neurology in Berlin, Germany using MRI imaging studies of the human primary somatosensory cortex found mirror-reversal in areas 3b and 1 in the third finger but not in the palm of the hand. When a subject performs a well learned motor act with the less preferred hand, it is unclear whether the reduced proficiency is due to control by a non dominant hemisphere which is somehow less capable or to interference by inappropriate motor commands from the dominant hemisphere from the same Wilkes and Sheely study of finger movements and handedness.

Studies of right handers and left handers state the strong right hand preference in humans remain a riddle; no lateralized behavior other than fine finger dexterity relates to it. Head turning consistency occurs towards the side with less dopamine asymmetry. Findings indicate that right handers prefer left sided turning and non right handers prefer right sided turning. Using the computer workstation with a computer keyboard with keypad on the left or the right will require head turning on each side. Will a dual keyboard and keypad based on your dominance require left and right head turning? Yes.

In cerebellum studies showing how both sides of the human brain are involved in preparation and execution of sequential movements, the cerebellum is bilaterally recruited for the preparation and execution, but activation in the primary motor cortex is restricted to the execution phase and most prominent in the contralateral hemisphere. In the Turkish Online Journal of Educational Technology, October 2002, Professor Dr. Emel Riza Almakhzoumi writes about brain activities and reminds us there are close relationships between brain activities and educational technology. The professor states there is a growth spurt of the brain between the age of 5 and 7 years. PET scans illustrate the different areas of the brain during activities involving language such as hearing words, seeing words, speaking words, and generating words. These scans show a difference in auditory stimulation resting states and the same with language activity, hearing, seeing, speaking and thinking. There are many studies by

NIH using magnetic resonance imaging and nuclear scanning techniques in both healthy and non healthy individuals.

In a study of motor circuits and handedness during finger movements differences are highlighted in the functional organization of motor areas in right and left handed people. The discrepancies that might reflect differences in the network features of motor system could also determine differences in motor activity that occur during recovery from injury. In the "Two Mind Theory" in how the brain is organized, visualize the right hemisphere is under left hand control with music, fantasy, art, creativity, genius, perception, emotional expression and a holistic thinking mode. Then for the left hemisphere under right hand control is language, writing, logic, mathematics, science with a linear thinking mode.

Different parts of the brain take care of initiating fine motor movements and also for gross motor movements. Geschwind's studies related histories of patients that could, on command, stand up, turn around twice and sit down but could not, on command, clench a fist. Brain organization studies show handedness and sidedness is apparent in brain scans and show differences between the right and left hemispheres. As you read this book and especially the research associated with handedness, brainedness and such, you will begin to understand the power that is in your hands. In a subscription I receive "World Science Net" in September 2009, their explanation is "Cities work much like brains, study finds: Highway interconnections in cities are organized and evolve much like brain connections, research suggests. http://www.world-science.net/othernews/090905_cities-brains."

## COMPUTERS AND PEOPLE, MEMORY, MIND AND SOUL

To continue my interview with Jeff Danick

*Grafton:* Now is a good time to bring in a discussion of how brain organization and the computer organization of hardware and software have similarities and disparities.

*Danick:* In my first example, of how thoughts or data move through different parts of the brain, you can look "Networking" on a very small scale. Looking at how different parts of an individual computer are "networked" together. On the surface, it seems similar, inputs and outputs, stimulus and response. However, the human mind is far more advanced. For any of the functions of the computer to function, you need software to control the hardware.

Two distinct things make the computer function as a computer, managing the inputs and outputs, the stimulus and response. We don't think of the mind that way. Well, some do, when you begin to discuss theories about what would happen to your soul if you had your brain put into another body. Would your soul remain with your body? Or would it go with your brain to the new one? But in terms of day to day living, most of us don't begin to partition our mind apart that way. Our mind is our mind, our brain and soul as one thing, a whole, us. Looking at how data moves through the mind and how data travels over networks of computers is also interesting. If we looked at each part of the mind based on their functions, what we know of them at least, and compared that to how data travels over networks between computers, we see some similarities. Technology still hasn't caught up to how adaptive the brain is in routing those signals. Remember, our brain cells are dying and being replaced daily. Our brain manages to route and reroute the data from all of our sensory experiences, the inputs and outputs, as well as the basic functions our body needs to survive such as regulating our body temperature and our heart rate.

*Grafton:* Continue with networking, please.

*Danick:* In the world of computers, when part of a network fails, more often than not, traffic on the network stops. One area that has begun to push that aside, is file sharing on the Internet. P2P applications like Bittorrent, allow someone to download one file they want from multiple sources at once. If one source fails, because the others are still available, the download continues. The software constantly searches for additional sources, and once the file has finished downloading to the user's computer, it becomes a source for others to download the file as well.

*Grafton:* What are your thoughts on memory and technology?

*Danick:* Memory and how our mind uses its "network" to find data in itself is where we are beginning to see advances in technology. Computers can store libraries of data on their hard drives, nothing new. Where it's beginning to get exciting is when you compare how we access old memories, old data in our minds. We may forget some things, but the important things, no matter how far back in our memories, and how many brain cells have died, are still reachable. The Internet, essentially and very large network, is beginning to give us that kind of access to data. Even when a web site has been changed, you can go to the internet way back machine web site, enter the web sites address you wish to view an older version of, and have access to years of past versions and revisions of websites and data. You can also access data on websites that are overloaded by looking at its Google Cache. Google, can, and does, cache some sites data, allowing you to view information that may be temporarily unavailable at the time from its original source.

*Grafton:* What are your thoughts on memory and the mind?

*Danick:* If you take the discussion of memory and the mind a
step farther, and look at how we can access memories, data
in our minds from a sound, or a smell, that type of recall
based on peripheral parts of the memory, we are seeing
developments in that area in technology as well. The next
version of MacOS X, 10.4, or Tiger, will include an
advanced search tool built into the OS that will allow you
to search your hard drive, or hard drives in other computers
on your network, based on "meta-data." In MacOS X 10.4,
you will be able to search for the word Jeff, and have: all
documents created by the user Jeff, all documents with Jeff
in their name, all documents with Jeff in their content, and
even all the contacts in your address book with Jeff in them
appear in an orderly list.

As you can tell Jeff Danick understands computer and networking very well. Danick can also spell out deficits in software and
ideas for developers to make headway. I have read in numerous
newsletters and websites, regardless of length of exposure to computers, they are hazardous.

Richard Seifert, Vice President of Federal Initiatives for Key Ova-
tion, from Ergonomics Today, "The Department of Defense alone
attributes $600 million annually to Worker's Compensation costs,
35% of which can be attributed to injuries preventable by ergonomic devices."

In an interview with Dale Brown, Project Development Specialist, Brown stated he had been working with computers since the
early 80s. He and his teams develop cutting-edge automatic testing
technologies for the Marine Corps and work extensively with the

Joint Services. When I first discussed the patent and the ideas behind the development of a different keyboard based on a person's dominance, he was more than interested as the ideas expressed are a win-win for all parties.

*Grafton:* Who are these winners?

*Brown:* Many benefit; society itself benefits as the idea reduces human misery; the employer, or company, benefits as the employees thus realize higher productivity, and indirectly increased corporate efficiency.

*Grafton:* How would you describe any differences between the human brain and the computer?

*Brown:* I have indicated how truly different the human brain and even the most advanced computers still are. The brain is an incredibly complex structure, quite flexible and subtle, capable of a seemingly astounding ability to adapt, create, and innovate on a scale not seen anywhere else on earth. The brain has been considered as possibly the most complex structure known, with some unsubstantiated speculation as to whether brain-specific quantum effects may be occurring within the depths of that very complexity. Additionally, the brain is capable of amazing deductive and problem solving capacities using only scant data."

*Brown and his son Eric have had many discussions on the nature of the brain. His sons' statement:* "the brain is quite possibly a *receiver* for the soul" puts yet another perspective on the matter.

*Grafton:* Where is computer technology going next in your opinion?

*Brown:* I have over twenty years experience working with computers but they still have a long way to go. Nonetheless, we have made incredible strides in computer technology by tireless efforts by numerous brilliant people in our basic understanding of both symbolic manipulations, the processing of information, and the hardware it becomes instantiated within. The latest technologies are pushing towards the realms of nanotechnology and quantum physics, opening up possibilities in the next decade or so that even within the laws of physics, that will try the imagination of even some of the most imaginative.

*Grafton:* What about software advances?

*Brown:* Software itself will one day become a seamless, 'augmented' reality with human-like interfacing-pushing state of the art flexibility. Right now, this software is still very primitive to what we will see one day. As an example, the Windows interfaces are too slow, it assumes we all think and organize in directory trees and folders. A future Windows-like interface needs to be far more intuitive and allow for a more richer and human-responsive environment. We live in a very rich, three dimensional, 360 degree visual world of infinite variety and texture with gargantuan amounts of information streaming about us. Yet we somewhat must constrain ourselves to a very small contrived world of our current computer paradigm. This must change, to better allow for human potential.

*Grafton:* Have you thoughts about the mind in education?

*Brown:* In the midst of this, in a time of unprecedented knowledge and discovery unlike any before known in human history, we stand on the brink of possibility and hope for a better future. We need to find ways to help us use this amazing gift of a mind we have, in ways such as to allow for a more complete expression of human capability and capacity. This includes conceiving new and innovative ways to adapt the computer to allow for human variation and potential to the fullest extent, rather than conforming the masses to the dictates of a cookie-cutter approach to computing, both in hardware and software. As in this innovative book, we need to seek multiple ways to free the mind, rather than corral it.

You may find it unusual for two people when asked about the inner workings of the brain and the computer to bring up the subject of the soul. The computer is quite simple and easy to figure out but not the human brain as no two people have the same experiences that add to the network of memories that foster our education. That education leads to the improvements in computer and software devices.

Plato's student, Aristotle, concluded the heart must contain the soul, and the brain's function was merely to cool the blood. The earlier belief by Plato included the theory that a perfect heaven rained down ethereal spirits that entered the body and were concentrated by the brain according to the Computer Continuum book mentioned earlier by Laukner and Lintner.

The Washington Post writer, Marc Kaufman, in the January 10, 2005 story about study and meditation wrote "mental discipline and meditative practice can change the workings of the brain and allow people to achieve different levels of awareness." According to W.M. Keck Laboratory for Functional Brain Imaging and Behavior "mental practice is having an effect on the brain in the same way golf or tennis practice will enhance performance. The brain is capable of being trained and physically modified in ways few people can imagine." He concluded his remarks with "scientists have embraced the concept of ongoing brain development and neuroplasticity."

Since two of the experts in computers mentioned what is lacking in computers is the soul? I could not help but fixate on the article by Diane Evans of Knight Ridder. The newspapers who asked "Where is the soul? How do you find it?" In this article "the physical action is necessary", "emotions" are needed, "purpose" and "complete faith" and "open" to new suggestions. When you hear the word soul, you may think more of spirituality. Spirituality generally entails a more inner directed and individual experience. For example, you can bring a creative force to your life if you can develop inner workings within your soul or spirituality.

In the new movie, What the Bleep Do We Know, the producers and writers bring out "the smallest form of consciousness-the cell" as their way to bring in nano technology and quantum physics.

## SOFTWARE KNOWLEDGE ACQUISITION

The famed inventor and MIT graduate, Ray Kurzweil, "periodically tracks 40–50 fitness indicators, down to his 'tactile sensitivity'." Not only is Kurzweil an inventor but a computer scientist and an author. Kurzweil's "interest in technology and health sciences" believe "all the genes we have, the 20,000 to 30,000 genes, are little software programs." Kurzweil also believes there will be a biotechnological revolution, in his book Fantastic Voyage: Live Long Enough to Live Forever.

Usernomics is a company that develops training programs and lists on their site, recommended books for the new age of computers. The website explains human factors had its origins in the Industrial Revolution and emerged as a full fledged discipline during World War II. In today's world, training programs must be easy to learn and easy to use. The Usernomics training program focuses on the user, not the product.

Rosilind W. Picard writes in her book, Affective Computing,

today's computers are cold, logical machines. She states computers must have emotion. "We must give computers the ability to recognize, understand and to express emotion." Brenda Laurel, in her book, Art of Human-Computer Interface Design, predicts the future direction of human computer interaction will have an overall relationship between computers and people.

In the search engine of your choice, type in nano technology and quantum physics and you will find how the computer and electronics with their chips are beginning to touch on memory. Can the hardware and software envelop the memory to produce sensitivity? There are others who say "the soul is infinite." Then will we live long enough for computer engineers and scientists in nanotechnology to develop these qualities? Are design engineers making computer networking more like human brain networking, or the other way around or is it a trade off?

An interesting study completed with stroke patients and the activity Virtual Reality received a comment from the lead author, Sung H. You, Assistant Professor of Physical Therapy at Hampton University in Hampton, Virginia, May 13, 2005. The five patients who took part in the study played the games, improved in walking, standing and balance. This progress was noted in brain scans before and after training showing reorganization of brain function after the therapy.

## ARTIFICIAL INTELLIGENCE DISCUSSED

"At every point in life, the brains plasticity (adaptability) gives us the ability to improve how our brain functions. It's only a matter of figuring out how to harness that remarkable capability" according to Dr. Michael Merzenich at Posit Science Corporation. Knowledge acquisition through use of the computer acquisition, retrieval and reasoning because production systems attempt to emulate the experts who write our software programs. Just look at Microsoft's Office Assistant. Searching is used when trying to create intelligent computers. The question would be, does the human brain use searching like the computer? No, but the concept of rules of thumb is used for more complex system developments.

Why is this important to you? By training in either the numerical data or mouse, you will show reorganization of your brain function after your training. Dexterity training for the average computer user will lead to the increase of brain networking within the individual computer user and will allow productivity in all areas of workforce innovation. You just may be the next person to revolutionize a hardware or software improvement from understanding and following up with the information in this chapter.

# CHAPTER FOURTEEN

*If you don't know how to do something, you don't know how to do it with a computer.*

**Source Unknown**

## MUSICIANS AND TYPISTS

In a study at the Biofeedback Institute of Denver, researchers were able to predict a subject's brain dominance by their choice of occupation. Musicians, athletes and artists were expected to be right dominants. Individuals in occupations with less structure (athletes, painters) were right dominants. Computer users and pianists use many of the same finger pattern movements. This may also be true of guitarists, violinists and others.

If you have access to a piano, please look at the keyboard. Apply this access to you as the computer user at the keyboard. Are keyboards just keyboards? How different are the machines (piano, computer)? Very different to be sure. But the people who operate these machines are so very different and all due to brain organization and past experiences.

## SIMILARITIES IN KEYBOARDS OF
## TYPISTS AND MUSICIANS

By looking at left handers websites, you will see many of your favorite entertainers in the music world are lefties. One can only wonder where else in these mixed handers or lefties are they superior? Sforza

C., Macri, Tirci, Grassee, Ferrario. (2003) in their study of finger movements during piano playing found that in "In both of them, the thumb was the most repeatable finger; in the girl, the fifth and fourth fingers scored the best repeatability." From other research, the thumb in pianists, guitarists and violinists received the most injuries and complaints for treatment.

In typing research and statistics between usages of the hands on the typing keyboard, the left hand is used 56%. After reviewing several beginners' piano instruction books, I knew I was on the correct path with my view of how to train the hands. Initial piano instructions begin with placing the right hand and start learning the chords left to right. Also placing the left hand to start learning the chords, right to left.

When comparing performance, Halinger (2004) in his biotechnology findings suggest increased efficiency of cortical and subcortical systems for bimanual movement control in musicians. "Using an MRI, they viewed parallel and mirror image sequential finger movements playing scales practiced daily by pianists and musically naïve controls. The naïve controls showed stronger activations within a network than pianists."

I have already mentioned video games players as not only prone to hand and finger injuries but also the same research areas apply. Eric Gwinn of the Chicago Tribune wrote "Author sees link between music, video games." Seth "fingers" Barcan was interviewed by him. "Jazz and video games are very similar" said Barcan. "He makes his fingers dance around." Making your fingers dance around the keyboard and keypad is an art for sure. When I took typing in college, my rate was 90 words a minute. I thought that was a fast speed. But in truth, skilled typists can type 130–140 words a minute.

In his book Mozart's Brain and the Fighter Pilot, Richard Restak, MD writes a large proportion of brain tissue is devoted to sensation from the motor power to the fingers. To further explain the power within the hands, Restak asks you "in your reading, pause and hold up one of your hands. Then rapidly touch the tips of each of the other four fingers to the thumb. With that simple gesture you have telescoped into one instant 50 million years of evolutionary development." Restak also believes one of the reasons of this is both the sensory and motor areas are exclusively dedicated to the hands. Restak also asks you "to remember that skilled musicians activate widely separated through interconnected areas by reading music and even just mentally rehearsing a musical score. At every waking moment, feedback exists between the hands and the brain."

## INTERVIEW WITH A PIANIST/TYPIST

I found that last statement to be true during an interview with a musician, pianist, singer and writer (typing and computer). Her background as a successful entrepreneur, performer of classical cabaret and popular music, and teacher of meditation who has created "Your Life Path", a life-enhancement system.

*Grafton:* When did you learn to play the piano?

*Arlene K:* I learned at the age of seven at my home from a Juillard trained teacher and have played throughout my life.

*Grafton:* Do you just play or do you teach?

*Arlene K:* I mostly play but I have taught and I am thinking about starting to teach again.

*Grafton:* Do you do any warm up exercises before you play the piano?

*Arlene K:* Yes, I do hand and finger warm ups at least fifteen minutes prior to playing but I recommend thirty minutes. I would do thirty minutes, but I get so impatient to start, I start and cannot wait to play.

*Grafton:* Do you have a name for the exercises?

*Arlene K:* Yes, the Hanon method. It is a very famous system of warm up exercises.

*Grafton:* Have you ever had any hand or finger complaints from piano playing?

*Arlene K:* No, but I was injured once and had fifteen fractures on my right side and was unable to use my right hand. So, I started to use my left hand to write and felt comfortable doing so.

*Grafton:* Are you right handed?

*Arlene K:* Yes.

*Grafton:* Are you right brained?

*Arlene K:* No, I would say I am balanced in my learning, speaking, playing and writing.

*Grafton:* Have you had any experience with or heard anything about computer use and Carpal Tunnel Syndrome?

*Arlene K:* Yes, I have read several articles about the problem.

*Grafton:* Tell me about your computer set up at home.

*Arlene K:* My chair is ok, but my lighting is not right. I feel I need to make some changes.

*Grafton:* I have reviewed what you do which is computer writing with no numerical data use and you are right handed, so I do not recommend my training techniques other than to check out the OSHA website eTool and review the equipment checklist. You already know specific hand and finger exercises.

*Arlene K:* Yes, I will do that.

*Grafton:* You have heard my message about exercising with a warm up routine prior to computer usage, would you recommend that to our readers?

*Arlene K:* Absolutely. I also recommend assessment of everything before you start anything.

## THE HANON METHOD

Following that interview, I searched the WEB for the Hanon Method and found several interesting sites with the information confirming again how similar the skills are between typing and piano playing. The New School of American Music recommends breaking "up the play session into four parts" fifteen minutes sessions if you are planning on an hour. The "first part of the session: warm up and exercises." They give two reasons for this: 1)"its pre arranged and repetitive", and 2)" after you have warmed up properly, you should be better able to play the rest of the lesson with fewer mistakes and more focus." They also recommend major scales and of course the finger exercises without the piano, just moving the fingers in minimal stretching and placement, similar to the piano finger movements.

This same web site shows one year's training starting with the first month, both right and left hand use learning both bass and chords. The second month, basic right hand techniques and the third month basic left hand techniques. In the eighth month, they bring in use of the metronome. Recommendations are to use the metronome as you go over your finger movements. "Start with a relatively slow count until you can master your drill, three times without error" before you increase your speed.

These teachers remind students, "training, the hand takes, no matter how fast you learn the material mentally." Famous pianist, Keith Emerson, in the article Emerson Unmasked, was once asked "in an interview about his practice regimen-he mentioned the old staple, Hanon." The article showed his practice scales "drawing singles bars ascending followed by a single bar descending." In other words, with the right hand scale left to right and with the left hand scale right to left.

Another piano teacher, Richard Beauchamp, writes there is "stress in piano playing." For prevention, Beauchamp recommends warm up the fingers before "stretching the fingers plus hot water warm up, smile" and "breathe while you are practicing and take frequent breaks." What do pianists do to avoid stress? "Do the Hanon five finger exercises." Beauchamp gives his reasons for stress as practicing too long without a break, too fast playing without allowing time to recover, working against the clock, posture and seating not correct, over clinching the fingers, or extreme positions of the wrists or fixed positions of the wrist. These are the same reasons given by OSHA, NIOSH and the BLS in their recognition of problem areas.

Professor and Artist Pianist, Huo Huang at Scripps College, recommends avoiding repetitive strain by learning to do neck rotations, side stretches and use shaking motions of the shoulders and arms as advanced swimmers do. Pianists need "agility and flexibility" not strengthening of the fingers. Cortol wrote exercises for the 3rd and 4th fingers, Brahms stretches for small hands and Lizst for power and speed, according to Huang. Huang states "if it hurts to play, you are not doing it right." So, whether you play piano or use a computer, keep those last few comments by Huang in mind as they certainly apply to both.

## MUSIC TO PLAY WHILE TYPING

As for the types of music to play while you are learning the numerical keypad training, I found a website "Leroy Anderson- Hear the Music." For starters, listen to the 1945 music from the "late show WLBS-TV in NY" for over 25 years, the Syncopated Clock. It is in 4-4 time. Gradually work into the Sleigh Ride, Plink Plank Plunk, Sandpaper Ballet, Jazz Pizzicato, and Fiddle Faddle and after you are really fast, try The Typewriter written in 1950.

Should you need more than this, consider a rhythm addition. The Finger Drum Mousepad sells for $39.95 at SkyMall. This device allows you to play eight different percussion sounds, including bass, snare, two rack toms, a floor tom, hi-hat, crash and cymbals only using only your fingers. You can also record up to 30 of your own rhythms.

In the book The Human Body and How it Works about coordination, the writer explains "models of learning (playing the piano for example) are produced by the cerebral cortex." These patterns "must undergo many rapid changes in response to variations required for the movements" of the fingers. These "models have to be learned and it is this learning process which makes necessary the long hours of practice to acquire the skills" necessary for excellence.

McManus C., Kemp, and Grant (1986) in the Cortex study of female pianists and typists and the "differences between fingers and hands in ability showed that separate mechanisms are inferred, and it is suggested that differences between fingers are a function of differential peripheral motor control, whereas differences between hands are a consequence of cerebral dominance of control mechanisms." Everyone's brain organization is different due to their life experiences.

You may think computer users and pianists are the only people that must learn to use both hands? According to a news article July 5, 2009, by Jeff Baenen for the Associated Press relates Billy McLaughlin, a fingerstyle guitarist is noted for his technique of tapping on guitar strings. But Billy began having problems controlling his left hand while playing, missing notes with no clue why. Billy was accused of being drunk. The culprit? Focal Dystonia. Billy received this diagnosis of the incurable neuromuscular disease. Did Billy quit his vocation? No. He learned to use his other hand. By switching hands and having his two guitars refitted and restrung for the left hand, he has received his first custom-made left handed guitar and is on tour in 2009.

You may be parallel/mirror image, or mirror/mirror image or parallel/parallel image in your handwriting test and/or finger circling test. It is ok, whatever the result. Work within your brain organization and increase your networking with using the left hand. I hope these studies and true life stories are as meaningful to you as to me and why I have gone to such great lengths to devise a way to help injured computer users.

# CHAPTER FIFTEEN

*The workers and professionals of the world will soon be divided
into two distinct groups. Those who will control computers and
those who will be controlled by computers. It would be best for
you to be in the former group.*

**Lewis D. Eigen**

## PERFORMANCE AND INDIVIDUAL DIFFERENCES

There are "two ways of measuring handedness, questionnaires and
hand-efficiency tests write noted researcher R.A. Rigal in 1992.
Rigal used "a method for combining performance scores of 128
children from different hand-efficiency tests to obtain a single handedness score based on efficiency." Rigal used "handedness classifica-
tions according to different thresholds of preference as well as of
performance." "To select pure right or left-handers, it is argued that
handedness should be established simultaneously through preference
questionnaires and performance tests and that only subjects falling
simultaneously into the same category on both measures are kept."
We can argue right along with all the researchers about advantages
and disadvantages of these two tests. But this is certainly a good
starting place.

## INTERMANUAL COORDINATION
## AND MOTOR LEARNING

Some of the tests used for hand skill are finger tapping, peg moving,
square marking, dotting or line drawing between targets or even
punching holes through targets. Gorynia et al. (2000) in their study

of intermanual coordination found higher values in intermanual coordination and reduced asymmetry in finger tapping may be associated with a greater bihemispheric control and better performance in fast bimanual movements.

In the Health Sciences, Motor Learning is a required course. Ullen (2003) in how movement sequences are processed independently provided evidence for the existence of independent systems for learning and representation of ordinal and temporal sequences and for implicit learning of temporal sequences. This may be important for fast learning and flexibility in motor control.

Numerous studies show tactile learning and motor control after stimulation of the right and left median nerve in the forearm increased the second somatosensory cortex to the right after a magnetometer stimulation but not to the left. Humans have control between the fingers of the right hand for sequence of learning as results showed that different sets of cortical regions are dynamically involved in motor sequence learning. McFarland (1975) found "when the left hemisphere is occupied by a verbal task, left hand performance by right handers improves."

The website Sharper Mind Centers indicate when determining direction, holographic directionality works much as the same as a computer does. Levy and Gur studied individual differences in psychoneurological organization and found that, as expected, writing requires access to the language hemisphere. Thus, "the dominant writing hand always appears to be under the control of the language hemisphere."

Individual writing styles have been studied by many disciplines. There are two different writing styles for left handers, straight writing style and the hooked handed writing style .According to Levy, there are two kinds of left handers, those with same-side neural dominance and those with opposite-side neural dominance. Levy contends that "people who have language in the left side of the brain yet write with the left hand must have access to those language centers in order to write." "There are only two ways they can do" that. They must use same side pathways or some form of relayed control of the commissures within the brain. Levy concluded the problem of left handers and language by saying there is "a majority of their motor fibers that fail to cross." The crossing is the corpus callosum.

## EYE DOMINANCE RESEARCH

Trembley believes every child should be tested for eye dominance when they begin school to make certain the left-handed child does not go against nature by writing right-handed when they should be left-handed. There are other writers/researchers who link disease with handedness. Trembley was noted for his books in aptitude testing.

Rapid finger tapping is a time honored task in the study of motor skills according to H. Heuer (1998), for example in comparing performance characteristics of the preferred and non preferred hand. Heuer is his study of "blocking in rapid finger tapping found that blocking affects the intertap by delaying the intervals by about twice their normal length." He concluded that the amount of time on task might increase the frequency of blockings in cognitive tasks."

Kimura and Vanderwolf (1970) found that both left and right handers showed a "superiority of the left hand on an individual finger movement task, but the difference between the hands was greatest for right handers." This leads to my observation and speculation that left handers and mixed handers would more easily learn the dual system from numerical data and mouse training.

In a laterality study, Bradshaw (1983) studied "hemispace." The corporeal space to the left or right of is the (usually body) midline regardless of, for example where the hands are placed. They tested subject's "when heads were tilted to the left or right, manipulated gaze direction to the left or right, and auditory listening coming from invisible loudspeakers." They "weakly confirmed the same findings of others of a left hemispace superiority though either hand was more accurate in its own hemispace."

Berner (1953), an ophthalmologist, studied the relationship of ocular dominance, handedness and the controlling eye in binocular vision for performance, states "the connection of the chain of difficulties with crossed dominants has long been noted." He concluded "during his investigation in over 500 patients with and without symptoms of reading difficulty, defects of speech and allied visual motor disorganization to form the following hypothesis:

When the controlling eye is on the side of the handedness no confusion is likely to occur.

When the controlling eye is on the side opposite the handedness some part of all the chain of symptoms is likely to occur.

When two hands are used the stronger the relative control of one eye if the controlling eye is on the side opposite the more commonly used hand, if the use of the second hand disrupts a well established eye hand pattern on the opposite side, symptoms are likely to occur."

When reading studies are measuring performance, left handedness and left footedness were strong predictors of slower reading groups. While Corac and Poren write about eye dominance as a part of generalized laterality, control of the limbs is basically a function of the contralateral cerebral hemisphere. Optic information from each eye reaches both cerebral hemispheres due to the partial descussating of the optic fiber at the chiasm. Their conclusion that males were more consistent in their sighting preferences than females is the general conclusion in performance studies of eyedness.

## GENETIC AND PATHOLOGICAL LEFT HANDERS

Because of our specific genetic inheritance, our family life, and our early training, most of us prefer to use one side of the brain more than the other. When one is forced into utilizing a weaker way of learning — or a new way — fear is evoked. This fear can be helpful to us in honing special talents or skills. The right brain is host to motor skills. As a problem-solver, it looks at the whole situation. The ideal person has strong skills in each hemisphere and can move into the appropriate one when that skill is needed.

The importance of individual differences is paramount to the reduction of stress associated with learning or relearning. As a worker, you need to know yourself well for peak performance at the office. Levy and Gur in their neurological studies looked at individual differences in psychoneurolgical organization and found that, as expected, writing requires access to the language hemisphere. Thus, "the dominant writing hand always appears to be under the control of the language hemisphere. They concluded it would not matter if the control pathways from the language hemisphere lead directly or indirectly to the ipsilateral (same) hand in others, to the contralateral (opposite) hand."

At the University of Indiana, M.K. Holder, writes about the Handedness Research Institute. There are basic problems with left handers in society. The bias is both intrinsic and socio-cultural that parents, educators, the medical community, employers and engineers must deal with product design.

Knecht, in the Brain, (2000) study of Handedness and hemispheric language dominance in healthy humans, that because of "atypical right-hemispheric language in left-handed patients" their conclusion "clearly demonstrates that the relationship between handedness and language dominance is not an artifact of cerebral pathology but a natural phenomenon." These are two opposing views from Levy and Knecht.

Another view was demonstrated by Vaid in Neuropsycholgia (1989) who studied "Hand dominance for signing." They counter "virtually all right handed individuals and left hemisphere dominant for language. Sign languages of the deaf provide an unusual vehicle for exploring the link between handedness and hemispheric specialization for language since in sign language the hands themselves are the language articulators." Their conclusions were "opposite patterns of asymmetries in hand performance were found in right and left handers. However, left handers were more flexible than right handers in signing with their non preferred hand."

Ornstein in his book, the Psychology of Consciousness, provided a clear description of the differences in information processing between the two hemispheres. He believes the right hemisphere function is obviously best suited for simultaneous and instantaneous processing of information required in sports.

Allen Bragdon and David Gamon in their book, Brains That Work a Little Differently, about recent discoveries and common brain diversities include left handedness as an atypical brain condition that can affect a huge proportion of the world population. There are genetic left handers who gain this trait from their family and those that are pathologic left handers, or those through some embryonic happening, before birth or during birth, or other accident early in life.

## DIFFERENCES IN LEFT HANDERS

Now that you know you have a dominant eye, have you noticed if you are left eyed and during the training, you found the left hand training easy? Noted researcher, Stanley Coren, asks Does Society Make Right Handers? Due to the fact of review of their studies, with less and less numbers of left handers that through the years, culture pressure makes right handers out of left handers. From our culture it is a learned response. Dr. Coren writes when we are talking about handedness and hand control, as many as twenty three brain centers and neural pathways are involved. These include several different movement control systems and position sensing systems that originate in the cerebral cortex.

Tankle (1983) studied mirror writing in right and left handers.

He found that movements away from the body are more accurate than movements toward the body. Tankle concluded from his studies there is a bias of writing learned from left to right. Lefties can more easily overcome the bias according to his conclusion. If you have never tried mirror writing, then get set for a quick lesson in frustration, as it is all new learning.

Orton is his studies concluded that lefties have left hemisphere dominance for language or a mirror engram stored and are better because they have direct access. This holds true with most researchers' conclusions. Norman Geshwind, a Harvard medical doctor states "the dominance organization is in the brain of left handed person is not like the majority of the population." Other scholars have studied verbalizer-visualizer questionnaires to determine dimensions of cognitive style.

These new ways of thinking have revolutionized creative teaching methods to assign in teaching to individual differences. Geshwind followed through on the research efforts of a group from Johns Hopkins University. They both proved that math geniuses may have a hormonal basis. In a report in Science Magazine (July 9, 1982, page 141) proposes "there is a link when mathematical genius occurs because mathematical ability is generally thought to be a right brain function." He states that "testosterone in fetal life gives the explanation why more boys are left handed than girls. This testosterone can alter brain anatomy so the right hemisphere of the brain becomes dominant for language-related abilities and the person is left handed."

## PSYCHONEUROLOGICAL RESEARCH

With the topics of performance and differences in people, you can see why I continue to bring up the subject of handedness and laterality. There is a side bias. The way to overcome this bias is to "engage in activities that stimulate extensive portions of the brain." These are more words from Dr. Restak. Typing or computer keyboard and keypad using is a whole brain exercise and requires you to use your powers of concentration.

Touch is an important factor in research too. Force, heat, cold are used frequently in motor learning to test learning. Stoeckel (2004) in his study of left and right superior parietal lobule concluded that "kinesthetic information is processed in the anterior portion of the superior parietal cortex with a right hemispheric predominance for discrimination and a left hemispheric predominance for information maintenance." The word kinesthetic means awareness or knowing, usually in reference to the five senses.

Grip force is used with the cursor but pressure from your fingers and feeling where your fingers are on the keypad or keys are sensory components for touch discrimination. But when you move your fingers, the motor components come into play. When I think about the senses, the concept of pitch comes to mind. If you compare, for example, the keyboard of the computer with keypad and the piano keyboard, the low notes are situated on the lower steps and higher ones to the top or the more conventional low at the left and high on the right. That is how both the piano keyboard and the numerical keypad are set up. Generally with touch, you also think of texture or how does it feel? I have been unable to find evidence that different keyboards (piano or computer) have a different texture. There is a little difference with force in typewriter typing and computer typing.

In an interview at the music shop of Michael Mancini, this self described musician player who is in his eightieth decade recalls some of the great days of the Big Band era.

*Grafton:* When you are playing an instrument, do you focus at all on how much pressure you put on the parts?

*Mancini:* It depends on the quality of your instrument. If you have a high quality instrument, you use a very light touch.

But if you have a low quality instrument, this will require a firmer touch or pressure.

*Grafton:* Do you pay attention to where you place your hands when you play?

*Mancini:* I know more about saxophones, clarinets and flutes. On these instruments, you must place your left hand on the upper half section and use your right hand for the keys.

There is no other way to do it.

In a discussion with Jay Agnew, Technology CEO.

*Grafton:* Do you use any different touch pressure from the usual computer keyboard and your lap top keyboard?

*Agnew:* I do not notice anything different except on my lap top. I use my thumbs more and use so much pressure that my office worker came in one day and said, what are you doing? Pounding on your keypad or what? I did not notice anything different until she came in and told me that.

Three reports from the May 2005 issue of Science Daily News were of interest to me. At the Howard Hughes Medical Institute study of October 26, 2000, researchers "identified a protein molecule that may play an important role in sensing delicate touch. By deleting the gene BNC1 greatly reduces the ability to sense light touch. When a hair is touched, receptors near the hair fire, triggering a nerve impulse that signals the hair has been moved. The sense of touch is not as well understood at the molecular level primarily because it is difficult to study the tiny nerve endings that sense touch."

The John Hopkins new lab could help robots "feel" more human.

If robots are going to have a sense of touch to go with sight, hearing and smell, someone needs to build "fingers" for them. Also the engineers in the Virtual Reality Laboratory at the University of Buffalo have developed a new technology that transmits the sensation of touch over the internet. The new technology is called sympathetic haptics and holds much promise as a teaching tool.

One of the more important writers and researchers in force and the hands is D. M. Rempel. One of his studies with others at the University of Michigan investigated applied forces using alphanumeric keyboards. "It was found that the peak forces corresponding to each keystroke were 2.5 to 3.9 times the required activation forces, indicating that the subjects consistently displaced the keys to their limits." In another study of carpal tunnel pressure during hand maneuvers "during typing the pressure rises baseline and remains elevated as long as typing continues."

## BIOMETRIC TECHNOLOGY

Biometrics is the new wave of identification used by security officers: fingerprints. Automated teller machines use iris recognition. Active signature recognition or the electronic pad reads the speed, pressure and direction of the writer's strokes as we use our credit cards. Braun in Germany studied "The right hand knows what the left hand is feeling." These researchers explain "The mislocalization profile, the incorrect localization of faint tactile stimuli to different regions of the body, has been shown to provide insight into the processing of tactile stimuli." "Interhemispheric somatosensory processing was examined in 15 subjects by studying the interference of left-hand stimulation on right-hand perception. In different conditions suprathreshold interference stimuli were applied to the left thumb or little finger either 200 or 500 ms prior to the application of a test stimulus on the right hand. Data show that interference stimuli applied to the left hand massively altered localization responses for stimuli applied to the right side. Stimulating the left thumb yielded an increased number of mislocalizations to the right thumb. Similarly, stimulating the left little finger caused a shift in localization responses towards the right ring finger. Results support the hypothesis that interaction of somatosensory information originating from different sides of the body follows a somatotopic organization."

What I envision within the networking of the computer and the computer user is a read out of energy within the nerve endings of the fingers as they are placed upon the keyboard. Just as finger printing, voice, facial, DNA matching and eyes are used as passwords now, sensitivity must be the next step. This should have an effect upon flight simulation in the future.

If you use both types of computer keyboards, you may need to check on the difference in touch pressure from keyboard to keyboard. And there will be differences in how each individual's brain organization in those segments relate to your ability to learn. Eliassen (2000) at the University of California at Davis Center for Neuroscience studies simultaneous bimanual movements of the hands and fingers. His study, "specifically, callosal transmission affects the degree of bilateral synchrony with which simple simultaneous hand and finger movements" are initiated. What was interesting about this study was the "changes suggest that anterior and posterior callosal fibres may make unique contributions to bimanual synchronization, depending on whether responses are self-initiated or in reaction to a visual stimulus." This study "demonstrates that neural communication across the fibers of the corpus callosum strongly influences the temporal precision of bimanual coordination."

Hager (2000) in his study of human finger movements comparing digits, hands and movement frequencies concluded that "movements of the thumb, index finger and little finger typically were more highly individuated than were movements of the middle or ring fingers. Fingers of the dominant hand were not more independent than were those of the nondominant hand." These researchers believed that "simultaneous motion of noninstructed digits may result in part from passive mechanical connections between the digits, in part from the organization of multitendoned finger muscles and in part from distributed neural control of the hand."

Kimura (1970) found that right handers perform paired finger flexions more easily with their left hand with results pointing to superior fine motor control in the left hand. Treffner (1996) using a metronome to determine left and right rhythmic components provides insights into the elementary synergy between the limbs, the dynamical mechanism that modulates it and the nature of the asymmetry in left handed and right handed individuals.

Wessel (1997) in his study of self paced versus metronome paced finger movements evaluated by PET scans using a series of finger opposition movements concluded that "self paced movements are mediated by the supplementary motor area whereas externally triggered movements are mainly affected by the lateral premotor cortex." Thus, the posterior supplementary motor area and right premotor area appear to be related to the bimanual coordination of finger movements.

Just knowing your dominance and individual differences between your hands and fingers should make you more comfortable in the surroundings of your computer worksite. Have you found a difference in your finger exercises easier to do with your left hand/fingers than your right/hand fingers?

You will see in this book the handwriting or Torque Test used by T. Blau and also Franz et al., similar circling tasks used. Franz (2003) in his study asking "does handedness determine which hand leads in a bimanual task?" Their study tested on a bimanual circle task that required "drawing either in the same direction (parallel) or in a mirror symmetrical coordination mode with the two hands. The pattern of results was similar for left and right handers on parallel tasks, but group differences were found with respect to mirror symmetrical tasks." At odds with the general claim that the dominant hand leads, the present results indicated that hand dominance does not generally determine which hand leads.

Three other studies of bimanual movements concluded the theory proved the motor systems controlling each hand are prone to neural cross talk: errors on the tone counting task were significantly higher during asymmetrical circling than symmetrical circling but only at the transition movement frequency suggesting results that cognitive processes play a role in maintaining coordination patterns with regions of instability. As movement differences were patterned with the use of a metronome deviations from the circular trajectories were most prominent for movements of the left hand. Start thinking about how to relax yourself as you work with your new skills. You will need relaxation between the hands to accomplish your new goals. Both in motor dominance and finger circling skills, a metronome may be helpful to you.

## MALES AND FEMALES RESEARCH

Amunts (2000) in the study of interhemispheric asymmetry of the human motor cortex found a difference in males and females. "Male infants lack the larger connectors between the brain's hemispheres therefore messages are routed and rerouted to the right brain producing larger right hemispheres. This size advantage accounts for males having greater spatial abilities. No interhemispheric asymmetry was found in females." Thus, anatomical asymmetry was associated with handed ness only in males, but not in females, suggesting sex differences in the cortical organization of hand movements.

Nalcaci (2001) in his study of the relationship between handedness and fine motor performance was to "re-investigate the relationship between handedness and asymmetry in hand performance and if there is sex difference in motor asymmetry. In the total sample, the correlation between hand speed and the handedness score indicated that the distribution of hand preference is associated with left hand speed, but not right hand speed. Results also confirmed that right handed females tend to have more asymmetric motor function than right handed males."

Much research is being reported but the basis for understanding the results are unknown. For example, Gur (1982), from the University of Pennsylvania, in his study of Sex and Handedness Differences in Cerebral "Blood Flow During Rest and Cognitive Activity" concluded that "the direction and degree of hemispheric flow asymmetry were influenced by sex and handedness." They along with others consistently document their sex differences but the neurophysiological basis is unknown. In this study "using an inhalation technique, they measured 62 normal healthy volunteers aged 18 to 26. The sample included 15 right handed males, 15 left handed males and 17 left handed females."

As early as 1927, Downey studied dextrality types and their implications. He concluded that "in no investigation should the possibility of sex differences be overlooked, nor the probable existence of pathological as opposed to a natural left handedness." When I asked Mathew Monroe, computer programmer, of their over 100 employees, could he notice any difference in how the women were learning as compared to men? His reply of the two women he noticed, they picked up the techniques needed for graphics and were both mirrored individuals and they did not have a sports background. He only knew they were both productive early on. For an understanding of women and jobs and pointed job information in the coming years you can log on to the DOL website.

# PART SIX

## ONLY YOU CAN MAKE A DIFFERENCE

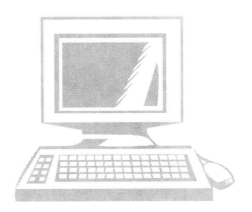

# CHAPTER SIXTEEN

*A distributed system is one in which the failure of a computer you didn't even know existed can render your own computer unusable.*

**Leslie Lamport**

## HAND AND FINGER MOVEMENTS

Earlier in the book regarding discussion about finger, hand and wrist movements, I named circumduction as a muscle movement. When we discuss direction or directionality in movement, you are required to use circumduction which is explained in the next study, of great importance in research and your understanding. Wilke (1979) in the "analysis of preferred direction of movements showed that strong right handers tend to move both left and right index fingers in the same direction and familial left handers tend to move them in opposite directions. Their study results indicate that interhemispheric interference in a motor skill consists of activation of inappropriate muscles of the non preferred hand by the dominant ipsilateral (same) hemisphere as its attempts to force that hand to conform to the direction of movement preferred by the dominant hand."

## IMPORTANT STUDIES

This particular study supports the view of this writer and researcher/ inventor why the dual keyboard and keypad based on dominance is needed to decrease the potential hazard of keying tasks by computer workers by the non preferred finger sequencing movement

179

through use of the keypad.

Grafton S., Hazeltine and Ivry (2002) explained the "human right hemisphere is active during execution of contralateral hand movements, and the left hemisphere is engaged for both contra and ipsilateral movements, at least for right handed subjects. Learning with the left hand also recruited a widespread set of temporal and frontal regions suggesting that motor skill learning with the non dominant hand develops within both cognitive and motor related functional networks." In this study using PET scans and the right hands of participants "the stimulus sequence and series of response locations remained unchanged, but the finger movements were different." This is why I use both fingers for circling and handwriting directionality measures.

**THEORIES OF HAND FUNCTION**

Finger tapping trials are one of the more common research techniques. In his book, Stanley Coren, writes about the inconsistency of the preferred hand or the better hand. Coren believes the most "interesting inconsistency between handedness and the agility of the hands is found in some forms of finger movements." "The ability to flex individual fingers seems greater in their left hand than in their right."

To test Coren's theory "bend the middle finger of each hand so that it forms an exact right angle while keeping the other fingers straight." Then "try to bend just the ring and small fingers into a right angle again keeping the other fingers straight." Then Coren asks you "move the fingers of each hand so that a V-shaped separation is opened between the middle and ring fingers." Coren's opinion is "right-handers find that these actions are usually done more easily with the left hand, but left-handers find the results less consistent." You may need to re read this paragraph and try these finger movements several times to make this more meaningful to you.

There are studies indicating a transfer effect when switching from one hand to the other. Kumar (2004), at the Indian Institute of Technology, Kharagpur, India, studied Motor performance as a function of verbal, nonverbal interference and handedness using finger tapping. He used both right handed and left handed humans in their trials. They summarized their findings as "Verbal as well as nonverbal interference conditions, as compared to non-interference conditions, significantly impaired finger-tapping performance of the left relative to right handers." Since you are not sure how your brain's inner workings are with verbal prompting, try it both ways while you are learning left hand usage..

In studies of hand and finger movements in the motor cortex regions in the brain found different areas were activated during same hand movements is spatially distinct from that identified during opposite hand movements. Hoffman G., Chang and Yim (1997) in their study of "student-use computers showed that 100% had the mouse installed on the right side." In this study of "moving the cursor to targets, as expected, left handers were superior to right handed users when using their non preferred hand."

## DOMINANCE AND SUB DOMINANCE
Researchers have demonstrated that hand dominance, handedness and type of movement influence different proportions of the brain. Brain activations are differentially sensitive to subdominant and dominant hand movements. Most researchers agree manual preference and skill are related. Annett G., Turner and Hudson (1974) in their study of the difference between the hands in motor skill "concluded it is difficult to answer the questions of the origins of difference between the hands in skill." "How much is due to difference in innate endowment and how much is due to the effects of practice are difficult to answer."

## PILOTS, CAD OPERATORS AND GAMES
People like to use the computer for learning. Computers can teach

just about everything. Generally these three categories are in group education and training: cognitive learning, psychomotor skills and social interaction. The relationship between the brain and muscles is termed psychomotor skills. Can you develop hand-eye coordination and rapid response with computers? Yes. Astronaut training for maneuvering of space craft and arcade and video games are instructional. If you look at video game players, or if you play, you will see that you must be well coordinated between the hands and fingers to be successful.

Finger tapping is required generally with both hands to move the game figures on the screen. The Nintendo games with the left hand side have up, down, left and right movements. But up is down and down is up. Go figure that one. The Game Boy control is built for the screen showing right hand players or left hand players. With a switch on the top left side of the control box, you can change the player to a left handed player. But this does not help the left handed player as the direction toggle stays the same according to a left handed video games player interviewed. But, the Intellivision II and Sears Tele Games Super Video Arcade have a Hand Control for each player. There are two actions buttons on each side of the Hand Controller. The top buttons, one each side, performs the same function for the convenience of either right or left hand players.

With so many youth fascinated with online gaming, a new report from PricewaterhouseCoopers predicts the numbers of online video game subscribers will more than quadruple between 2005 and 2009, as will online gaming revenues. The numbers predicted that online video game subscribers would hit 4.4 million in 2004 and are now 6.5 million. Should this keep pace several things could happen. Either youths' hand or fingers will be "worn out", will not last a lifetime, or computer work stations will have dual set ups for both mouse and numerical keypads to account for the increase of brain networking. Alarms have been raised about RSI in children and use of the computer and games. There is a website Kids Health for Parents with ways to deal with overuse of video games in children.

The video game industry can easily be measured by looking at the educational courses now offered by the Art Institute of Ft. Lauderdale, Florida, Miami Dade, Atlantic University, Keiser College, and Broward Community College as all see the relationship of what game developers want in the way of programmers. Schools are offering art and game design and programming and production. Many of the gamers and programmers are looking for fun jobs and the money is good. But, the concerns of risk on the job may be overuse of the hands and fingers as the hours are long. Florida is not the capitol of the games industry. California still holds that honor.

Gerloff C. (2002) studied bimanual coordination and interhemispheric interactions at the University of Tuebingen Medical School in Germany. "Bimanual coordination of skilled finger movements requires intense functional coupling of the motor areas of both cerebral hemispheres. They cite bimanual coordination is a high level capability that virtually always requires training and reflect the establishment of 'motor routines'."

To pilot an airplane requires high level coordination and an aptitude for fine motor control (hand and eye coordination). In a discussion with a Design Engineer for computer circuits, I explained to him my training method and believed the method had importance for the Department of Defense for pilot training.

*Grafton:* How could my product (training method) be of use for pilot training?

*Larry A:* I happen to also be a Pilot Instructor. In a two-seater, the joy stick is between the seats. If you are the pilot, sitting in the left seat using your right hand, you fly the plane with the right hand using the joy stick. The joy stick has certain movements that cannot be changed. You move the flaps one way, go up, and go down only one way. Now, if you change to the right side seat, you are required to use the left hand and that can be a problem.

*Grafton:* Now that you know you are a parallel learner with your handwriting test results, this would be easy for you?

*Larry A:* Yes, but for most people, it is difficult, so this is important for the aircraft industry to know, especially for two seaters.

A retired Marine Harrier pilot skilled in computer use had this to say.

*Grafton:* Now that we have talked about the joy stick and the two seater, what about computer controls in flight?

*Robert A:* Since most of today's aircraft have digital flight controls systems, there is certainly the possibility that you could include programmable flight controls as part of the digital flight control system.

*Grafton:* Explain that step by step.

*Robert A:* Each pilot could program the stick, throttle and HOTAS (Hands on Throttle and Stick) to control their respective systems in a manner that is best for that pilot.

*Grafton:* When would this be done and at what stage?

*Robert A:* This type of programming would be done during the pre-flight mission planning and could be specific for a type of mission and weapons load. One of the more common traumatic injuries for pilots are to the neck and caused from carrier landings and in time frequently cause hand and finger problems.

Two occupations that require drawing are Designers and Artists and the classes they take are Graphics Design and Technology and Design. With Graphics Design you may use Desktop Publishing, Photoshop, 3D, QT Virtual Reality and Multimedia, Computer Art, Digital and Studio Photography, Web Design just to name a few of possible software programs. Technology and Design courses include CAD, Drafting, Technical Drawing and other Construction type software. These types of workers must have fine motor control between the hands and the fingers.

In a conversation with an Architect about his CAD Operator's work station, he had this to say.

*Grafton:* How many systems does your CAD Operator use?

*Allen A:* I have watched my operator bring up at least four programs off and on very quickly, graphics, paint, drawing and others but he is so fast with his fingers.

*Grafton:* Does he use the right hand, left hand or both?

*Allen A:* He is a "righty", or at least he uses his right hand for all the programs. But for me personally, I use my mouse on the left hand side so I can write with my right hand. I get a lot more work done that way.

In another conversation with a Design Engineer for an equipment company.

*Grafton:* What are your experiences with CAD software?

*Brian C:* I have been out of CAD for nearly 10 years.

*Grafton:* What skills does a CAD user need to have?

*Brian C:* They need to be good at matching and have good visualization skills as well as good hand and eye coordination.

*Grafton:* Is a standard keyboard with keypad used for CAD?

*Brian C:* Yes, that is the standard set up here.

*Grafton:* Is it beneficial to be left handed for a CAD Operator?

*Brian C:* I do not know any left handers to make that judgment?

*Grafton:* Is there similarity in CAD software and graphics?

*Brian C:* CAD software is for mechanical drawing. Graphics would be of benefit for photos as in Marketing.

*Grafton:* Would a dual set up like Programmers be of benefit for CAD Operators?

*Brian C:* When I worked on CADAM, we have a dual setup with a function key pad to my left and a light pen I used on the screen. It was fine at the time, but the advancement of mice has more than made up for any benefits that system may have had.

*Grafton:* Tell me about your CAD Operator software?

*Brian C:* Our drafters usually have five software systems running all the time, CAD, MS Word, Explorer (to check the internet), ERP/MRP system and the on-line calculator. Their hands and fingers are busy.

The Graphic Artist who designed my patent drawings had this to say.

*Grafton:* Tell me about your computer work station set up?

*Ray D:* I have a regular keyboard, I am left handed and I have taught myself to be ambidextrous. I can draw with either hand with the use of the mouse and have a dual set up. It works for me.

For the serious photographer the Wacom Graphics Tablet along with the Intuos3 Grip Pen that reduces grip effort by 40% and the Intuos3 Five-button Mouse has five programmable buttons plus a scroll wheel, cordless and most of all "its ambidextrous low-profile design." "By alternating between the pen and the mouse reduces repetitive motion."

Apple, IBM and Microsoft are just three of the big players in the development for individuals with dexterity difficulties and impairments for the IT industry. Virtual reality simulation games and intellectual tutoring by medical device makers and the Department of Defense contractors will enhance their contributions in the coming years through use of my patent. I envision more product compatibility with human computer interaction researchers and ergonomics leaders will be proud of; continuing to make the study of fitting the job to the person, rather then the person to the job. Training both hands for the computer workstation will reduce the numbers of computer related repetitive strain injuries through time rotation with the hands and fingers from the right side to the left side leading to the custom dual workstation saving your hands, your fingers and increase productivity.

The training of the hands is very important for many of the occupations mentioned earlier in the book. In the coming chapters, I will continue to bring into your thought processes many of the human factors that will come into play in your training tips of how to better use your left hand, which may or may not be your preferred hand.

# CHAPTER SEVENTEEN

*The sad thing about artificial intelligence is that it lacks artifice and therefore intelligence.*

**Jean Baudrillard**

## ALL ABOUT LEARNING

In an earlier book, this writer recommended we should test adults and children to determine their best learning styles. Then to choose the appropriate teaching method to insure that all people can learn both visually and verbally. In this three step process 1) train both hemispheres, while allowing and reinforcing natural hemisphere development, 2) train students to use the cognitive style suited to the task at hand, and 3) train students to be able to bring both hemisphere styles to solve a problem in an integrated manner. Computer software companies are now using the term "Intellectual Tutoring."

## LEARNING STYLES

When reviewing students that are not doing as well (not learning), then determine if a visual or a verbal learner. A visual learner will close their eyes. A verbal learner will repeat verbally instructions, step by step. Which one of these actions helps you?

Alexander (1997) in the CIJE publication on teaching computer ergonomic techniques to secondary and postsecondary educators "found that more secondary teachers thought computer training should begin at the elementary level: they were more likely to teach about computer use hazards."

Through the development of computer use at early ages at home at school, Clancey (1996) wrote a booklet about "the increased risk of developing a repetitive strain injury." Clancey discussed RSI, CTS and "the increased incidence due to poor posture, poorly designed workstations and poor keyboarding technique."

Evelyn Hall at the Louisiana University studied hemisphere dominance and how to use your right brain. She concluded "very often the dominant left brain over rides the processing of visual and kinesthetic information inherent in movement." Hall states that "relaxation training and visual imagery techniques can increase the performer's ability to use the right hemisphere function to the fullest potential in sports. The greater shift to the right hemisphere control can allow a state of mind which yields stress free information processing in the appropriate hemisphere for movement."

Are you concerned with the slowness of learning with the left hand? Do not be as Peters J. and Ivanoff (1966) explored the role of handedness and computer mouse experience in cursor control performance. They found "specific hand experience dictated performance asymmetries, yet overall movement time differences between the practiced hand (usually the preferred) and the unpracticed hand was less than 0.2s." That is good news.

Should I do my training in the morning or afternoon? Boadella J., Sluiter and Frings-Dresen (2003) in their study of reliability of upper extremity testing found that a time effect in coordination tasks: keyboarding performance was better in the morning. Will a metronome really help me with training? Whitall (2000) in her study of bimanual finger tapping consistency and coordination found that tapping to a metronome had a differential effect on in phase and anti phase. If you are having rhythm and timing problems associated with training in the numerical keypad, I recommend a metronome.

## LEARNING SYSTEMS

The original findings were affirmed for preferred frequency. Nord E. (2001) used an operant conditioning program to train injured workers to control their muscles during work activities and provided support for this approach and justification for controlled clinical trials. He believed that work related upper extremity disorders continue to present treatment and financial challenges to providers, employers, and insurers.

Drawing on the Right Side of the Brain author Betty Edwards' teaching method is designed to reduce the amount of left hemisphere involvement in the drawing process. Her book is a stimulating view how important the eyes are in figure ground use or how you can manipulate what you see.

A simple way to outsmart the left brain is to know how to get to the right brain, your intuitive side, not the logical side. The easiest way is to find a small object on the wall in the room. Look at the object intensively, which is the figure. Then quickly look at everything around the figure, which is the ground and you will have accomplished the so called "cognitive shift." You can do this also with "other hand writing" as described by Betty Edwards in her works of creative learning. The author uses biofeedback, guided visualization and sensory stimulation too.

Will music help me with my training of the left hand? Springer and Deutsche, authors, indicate you can teach/educate according to the hemispheres. Their review of boosting right hemisphere thinking or training the right hemisphere is based on the over riding of the dominant right hand, left brain. Our custom of a sequential seeming world education wise would indicate we need development of the right brain. This can be done by playing music in the background to occasionally drown out presenting verbal information.

DeRosa A. (2004) state acquisition of new learning is challenged by the phenomenon of proactive interference which occurs when previous learning disrupts later learning. Their results with humans provide evidence for parallel neural systems, each with the potential to resolve interference in the face of competing information.

Neural networks of motor control are well understood and the motor domain therefore lends itself to the study of learning according to L. Muller (2002). He believes there is conflicting evidence for early and advanced stages of learning from their neuroimaging studies. In this study conclusion there were differences in visually driven explicit digit sequence learning during early stages and low performance.

M. Nadler (2000) in his study of acquisition of a new motor skill from finger muscles (index and little finger) investigated possible reorganization of central nervous pathways of the non dominant hand. His findings suggests that "learning a new motor skill produces changes which take place predominantly in the cortical pathways of the cutaneomuscular reflex and may be due to changed connectivity within the motor and/or sensory cortex." The study of the "neuropsychological processes behind learning, memory and perception are concerned with the neural events underlying such diverse phenomena's as motor skills, perception, motivation and learning."

## MIND STYLES

"Mind styles" are very important to teachers. The Myers/Briggs personality test is a widely used test by managers of people. The test divides people into individual preferences: Thinking-Feeling, Extrovert-Introvert, Judging-Perceiving, Sensing-Intuitive.

Charles G., a software and hardware computer trainer for a large USA company, travels to all parts of the northern hemisphere introducing new and upgrades for improved software use for new employees in the hotel industry. What was important during this interview unfolds.

*Grafton:* I asked the question, do you look at individual work-stations?

*Trainer:* Yes, and I would certainly say something if I saw anything out of line. You can tell whether they are confident or unconfident. Also you need to look at their age, as frequently the older learner is not as "hip" to computers. Then on the other hand, when you see someone in their twenties, they probably have been brought up on computers. For the older learner, take more time; go slower, step by step. On the younger learner, progress will be faster.

*Grafton:* What is special about your type of position?

*Trainer:* One of the more important issues for me is what is their job? By understanding what their job is, then focus on those essentials that are important for their job. Knowing your preferences and learning about other peoples can help you understand where your special strengths are, what kinds of work you might enjoy and be successful doing, and how people with different preferences can relate to each other has been valuable to society in general.

Learning systems are 1) rote, 2) instruction, 3) deduction, 4) induction, and by 5) analogy. Success in all levels of learning requires use of these systems. These types of learning are used in computer programs and are referred to as machine learning. Supervised training is the most common process for training a neural network, no matter the brain or artificial intelligence. No matter what you are attempting to learn, if you do not try to learn something everyday, your neurons will die. You must continue your learning so you can keep your brains' networking alive and interconnecting.

Biofeedback studies have shown that a human's short term memory is so very short: every eight seconds you lose about 30% of the sensations or feelings you have generated. That is, if no new ones have come along. So, concentration on the steps to learning to use the left hand is paramount. Your feedback is important too. Learning theory equates to immediate, accurate, reliable feedback with subsequent results. Do not allow confusion. Write down your questions in your log book or notes section for each page. Allow your actions with feeling which will fade from memory 30% every 8 seconds. Concentrate after each new step in your learning.

# CHAPTER EIGHTEEN

*The truth of a theory is in your mind, not in your eyes.*

**Albert Einstein**

## INVENTIONS AND IDEAS

The inventor for a dual programmable keyboard, Sanjay M. Patel "integrates conventional keyboard features to form a Multi-Dexterous Keyboard (MDK) system designed to minimize Repetitive Strain Injuries." It can be used as either a single or dual handed" providing "numerous ergonomic arrangements with simultaneous use as either a Left-Hand Side (LHS) or Right-Hand —Side computer keyboard module" and again, how do you know how to program the keys? Fentek Industries list an MCK-142 Programmable keyboard as $150.00 but a special of $125.00.

## SUGGESTIONS FOR KEYBOARD/KEYPAD LAYOUTS

How different is my patent and my training method? My idea is so unique in that it allows for different key layouts and device placement based on the user's preference to key placement and hand dominance for numerical input into computers and calculators. It can be used as a stand alone input device, or as part of a modular input system allowing placement of keypads with the differing layouts on the right or left of the users keyboard as needed, depending on the users hand dominance.

And what a difference in price? You can purchase an IBM 2-button PS/2 combo mouse on the web site www.TigerDirect.com for $2.99 while supplies last. Tiger Direct also lists the IBM/USB 1.1 Keypad/USB1.1 Hub, 17 key at a cost of $9.99. There is a difference in the MDK invention costs and my idea ($125.00–$13.00 for a saving of $112.00), so you may wish to take a look at your equipment checklist at this time before you buy.

The idea for an input device and corresponding key layout can be used for the numerical keypads featured in Windows/MacOS/Linux PC keyboards, as well as adding machines, also referred to as office machines and calculators. You may wish to review again the numbers locations and your work station set up for the explanation of numbers. Input devices used with PC's based on my idea should utilize USB connection technology and standard drivers for use with Windows, MacOS, and Linux based PC's. With the use of the new gestures system by Apple, you may just find these ideas have been formulated into the use of the Blau and Wilke-Sheeley tests in the keyboard and mouse section in the Control Panel on your computer. For the basic use of this concept, no special software should be required; however, special software could be used to aid in the training in the use of these input devices. Programmable keypads or keyboards require the inclusion of certain software applications to function well. You may need to go to the company's website to download any applications needed.

Keypad placement (left or right of user) and key layout (standard layout) or the mirrored layout. This should be changed by the user with ease based on their individual needs in an effort to reduce RSI that occurs with long term activity of this kind. Placement can be based on which hand they are more efficient with depending on task at hand.

A right hand user may prefer to use a mouse or other pointing device with their right hand while entering numerical data with their left. Depending on their hand dominance and other factors, they may be more efficient and incur less stress while performing the data input with the different key layout offered with this idea.

A left handed user may prefer to use a mouse or other pointing device in their left hand, while entering data with their right hand. Or, they may prefer to enter data with their left hand. A left hand dominant user may prefer the standard key layout on the left side, or the mirrored layout on the right.

In the case of adding machines, also referred to as office machines, or tape calculators, a left handed user may prefer the new keypad layout in this idea, which mirrors the typical layout found in most calculators. I have not seen anywhere is my research any office machines, programmable or not, different numerical directionality options for purchase.

Another system for the new learner in colleges, universities or other business schools would use the dual keyboard with the regular typing portion the same but with two numerical pads, one on each side. The new learner would learn at the onset of keyboard use the problem of overuse and repetition and this would relieve the situation in the years ahead for OSHA, BLS and industry in general.

In an interview with Russell Cameron, an experienced computer programmer, who not only is left handed but plagued by Carpal Tunnel Syndrome and all the discomforts of this in both hands:

*Grafton:* What do you think of my patent and training program?

*Cameron:* I see it as a method of teaching of ambidexterity.

*Grafton:* How do you see the difference in typing and numeric data entry?

*Cameron:* The biggest problem with typing and numeric entry is not allowing the wrist or arm to change position. I mean, support the arms at a comfortable width with some padding as there is a need to hold the arms in a comfortable position.

*Grafton:* Explain further.

*Cameron:* The nerve at the elbow gets irritated causing numbness in a couple of fingers first, then you get the wrists involved and both wrists and more of the fingers start to hurt. I personally have occasional pain in the elbow and almost constantly in my wrists.

Cameron has been working within the computer industry for more than twenty years and may need to leave the industry due to his disability. He has been wearing wrist splints at night for over ten years.

In studies of hand writing, the ability to write is a product of our way of life, which must be learned. Our way is left to right writing and reading. The Egyptians and Koreans use right to left reading and writing. This is a sensory motor process and you have read about this process in the research presented.

Following publication of this book, for large scale use, a computer program will be written to accomplish the same. A trial and error process could also be used allowing the computer or machine user a choice of which one is easier for them to coordinate their hands and fingers for data input. Also, I anticipate a video program will be developed to use in training programs at universities or schools for computer users in their initial learning experience.

## AN OVERLOADED SYSTEM
Many left handers have been taught to use the basic keyboard with the numerical portion on the right not the left. So there is a need to develop this system of keyboard design and educational efforts

to support this concept. The right hand side of the computer/keypad is overloaded.

Gene Dent, author of Return to Work....by Design discusses how internal programs are developed by businesses. He asks what department? Human Resources, Benefits, Occupational Health, Safety, EAP or even Risk Management. Ergonomic solutions don't need to be complicated, they can be simple. Quite possibly large companies with Ergonomic or Safety Officers would support the number of employees that have filed worker's compensation claims, then will have a need for these alternative keyboards and keypads with how to use videos for their safety programs.

In industrial accidents, companies look at the length of time or number of hours with repetitive use of the hands; right hand, left hand or both hands are generally on their accident forms. Often grasping and fine dexterity will also be listed. Companies are required by law to log in their injuries. When the logs are audited, they look closely at how many are injured for the same reason and what the company is doing to correct the problem.

Dr. Restak asks how you can "apply your knowledge about the human brain to organize your ideas." With the potential that every neuron in your brain can connect to the other, then why not begin to change your thinking and learn all you can. You will begin to see in detail why this simple use of your dominance can reduce the number of strain injuries from computer use or numerical data entry. If you have not done so, take a critical look at your workstation. Assess how you can make changes to reduce the strain on your arms, hands and fingers.

There is a multitude of data available from our government organizations. Computer users generally make 5% more salary than non-computer users from the statement 6/21/04 from www.bls.gov. Should you plan on continuing your occupation with computer use?

OSHA uses the word "preference" with left hand use with input devices. Preference is a choice. Dominance is genetic. Know what your dominance is, then select your input devices. Handwriting and gesture recognition and/or haptics for the two simple tests will be a boon for the developers for the assistive technology industry. The electronic industry will double their peripheral control devices of input sales as laptops are overcoming sales for the PC industry. Just as the Windows Operating System has applications for left and right mouse and direction of different languages, the new systems should have operating systems to include direction of the numerical keypad numbers rather than relying on keyboards for left-handers or keypads for left-handers. There is twice the number of women with computer related injuries.

By industry from BLS data internet services, data processing, information services, computer systems design and software publishers lead with growth rate of out put per year in 2002. Think now, how can I increase my productivity and longevity in the occupational position of my choice based on my genetic dominance.

# CHAPTER NINETEEN

*The cloning of humans is on most of the lists of things to worry about from science, along with behavior control, genetic engineering, transplanted heads, computer poetry and the unrestrained growth of plastic flowers.*

**Lewis Thomas**

## INJURY PREVENTION MEASURES

You will see and hear these terms in prevention: Safety, Ergonomics and Environment. In this chapter the topics for discussion are job demands, risk assessment, training solutions, productivity, and policy analysts. Human resource workers understand job descriptions and why this department falls into education and training of all employees. The Handbook of Disabilities states the CTS or RSI or CTD "is usually associated with a combination of poor job design." The handbook further states that "only 1% of individuals with CTS develop permanent damage from the problem." Individuals most at risk are "individuals using computers." The "avoidance of triggering activities-the treatment of choice" from the handbook. Possible functional issues are "difficulty with detail work involving hands or finger and difficulty typing." Too, 'career planning issues' must be developed and learning skills should be unaffected but "training or school is an option." "Ergonomic keyboards" are the "possible accommodations."

From research in Atlanta OSHA offices, repetitive injury, carpal tunnel syndrome, tenosynovitis, overuse of hands, arms, fingers are the largest users of lost time and worker's compensation benefits.

201

There is a need to develop services for customers to provide effective adaptive equipment. There is also a need for the educational system as persons are taught to use computers to know there are human factors related to their use and over use of keyboards. There is general information, ergonomics, organizations, resellers, alternative keyboards, accessories and other products available but not to the extent as explained in this book. We need to establish more effective return to work programs that give results with measurable outcomes for programs developed with use of prototype keyboards for right handed and left handed keyboard/keypad users. This also includes the mouse arrangement.

## TYPES OF LITIGATION

When a Workers' Compensation claim is made, frequently a litigated process is begun either by the claimant (injured worker), insurance company or the employer. There are many technicalities to these types of lawsuits. For example: from the website search engine West Law.1. "Kelly vs. NEC Technologies, Inc., Product Liability, August, 1992. New York. CTS, a form of RSI prevalent among keyboard users." 2. "Matter of NY County data entry worker product liability litigation, Aug. 17, 1994. The user alleged that her use of manufacturers' products caused her bilateral CTS." 3. "Berry vs. Boeing Military Airplanes, 12/9/94. Case of Bilateral CTS. Offers simplicity and establishes uniformity in the process in dealing with CTS." 4. "Bonquiorno vs. City of New York. Occupational disease had an earlier Workers' Compensation claim for back and neck injuries. An earlier claim where none of the doctors found a causal relationship between his CTS." 5. "Piper vs. IBM Corp. 1996. When symptoms developed into a diagnosable condition in her right hand, there was a three year limitation period." 6. "Depew vs. NCR Engineering and Mfg., Kansas, 10/31/97. Disability to be computed from the last day of work, one injury, that being CTS." 7. "Anderson vs. Boeing Co., Kansas in 1998. Our analysis to this point has demonstrated the complexities in fixing DOI (date of injury) or date of occurrence in a CTS case. CTS can cause permanent partial general disability." 8. "Hamilton vs. Dorka Industries, Inc. Tennessee 7/30/99. Rheumatoid Arthritis could very well be singular cause of M's. Hamilton's CTS. Dr. could not rule out whether RA has similar symptoms." 9. "Cozad vs. Boeing Military Airplane Co., 3/17/2000, Kansas. Employer knowingly hired handicapped worker with a pre existing CTS. Doctor probably would not have occurred but for pre existing CTS." 10. "SAIF Corp. vs. Chipman, Oregon, April 12, 2000. Computer input for major part of the day, computer keyboarding involves repetitive hand activity." 11. "Mulder vs. Liberty NW Insurance Co. Boise, Idaho, 9/29/2000. Sought benefits for medical expense associated with work related bilateral CTS, was an occupational disease." 12. "Brewer vs. Denver and Rio Grand Western Railroad, Aug. 28, 2001, Utah. Surgery both hands. Dr. advised him not to return to work to do that kind of work." 13. "Lanning vs. Virginia Dept. of Transportation, 3/26/02. Formerly worked at a toll booth, and then changed. Injury became worse due to constant use of the computer in her new position. The doctor explained how her prior and present work conditions resulted in injury, CTS."

To summarize, litigation can consist of disagreements of when the injury occurred, diagnosis was medically related and not work related, pre existing, prior work, date of injury, causation and of course product liability as mentioned earlier in the book. In July 2001, Labor Secretary Elaine Chao stated their new policy will put greater emphasis on preventing injuries and be based on the best available science.

The Keyboard Study by NIOSH was developed and is available at their website, www.NIOSH.gov. The Keyboard Safety Study by RSI an overuse injury association state that "winning your disability case requires three words, frequency (task), severity (injury) and duration (length of service). Now is the time to develop this dual system to reduce work place injuries. At the web site www.osha.gov The National Advisor Committee on Ergonomics met in Washington January 27–28, 2004. At this meeting "the committee will hear presentations at the research symposium." Also additional "topics related to the diagnosis of injuries and workplace ergonomics programs" will be heard. The name of this research symposium is Musculoskeletal and Neurovascular Disorders — The State of Research Regarding Workplace Etiology and Prevention." OSHA "estimates that work-related musculoskeletal disorders in the US account for over 600,000 injuries and illnesses that are serious enough to result in days away from work (34 percent of all lost workday injuries report the BLS)." "It is estimated that employers spend as much as $15–18 billion a year on direct costs" for these types of injuries.

As a result of the study of musculoskeletal disorders, NIOSH published "A Primer Based on Workplace Evaluations" which is another free service of our Government for dealing with musculoskeletal disorders. Looking for signs of work related musculoskeletal problems, setting the stage for action, training and building in house expertise, gathering and examining evidence of MSD, developing controls, health care management and proactive ergonomics is the basic information provided. There is also a tool box given for assistance in how to put a program in place to reduce MSD.

Injury prevention appears to be the wave of the future for these conditions. "HealthyComputing.com was founded in 1999 to address the growing problem of computer-related injuries." These disorders have been known in the past but "there is one major difference" "by using computers, we now are almost all at risk" according the www.rsi-center.com/. Companies that invest in safety consistently realize positive bottom line results. While you are on line, in the Search screen, type in the name of your computer and safety. All computer makers must adhere to certain guidelines and warn of the dangers of their particular computer.

Articles from The National Law Journal, February 25, 1995,

state they are "hoping stress injuries from keyboard use will become the mass tort of the 1990's." From the ABA Journal, February 1997, "In Madden v. Digital Equipment Corp., the jury awarded $5.9 million, $5.3 million of which went to one plaintiff who has lost the use of her left hand. Most keyboard injury trials have been decided in favor of the defendants, but hundreds of suits have resulted in settlements."

In their definition of health, The Hand, www.med.unc.edu, to understand RSI and to appreciate its significance, the magnitude, the impact "nearly half the US work force, some 60 million Americans, use computers on a daily basis or at home" and "keyboard users are emerging as a significant segment of the RSI afflicted work population."

What happens if you are a computer user, having symptoms of RSI, MSD or CTS? After conservative treatment several times, then surgical evaluations are often requested. Surgery is not always the answer either, as second surgeries are frequently performed. Many studies point to "surgery is the definitive treatment for CTS" according to South African researcher, rgraham

According to the CTDNEWS May 17, 2004, "More than 25,600 CTS surgeries performed in single year" from the neurosurgeon report. There are other surgeons that perform CTS surgeries too, i.e., orthopedic surgeons. "Surgery for CTS alone can cost $30,000. Not including efforts at retraining, benefits, time off and litigation costs" according to the www.med.unc.edu website.

**INTERVIEWS WITH COMPUTER USERS**
One of my referrals for an ergonomic evaluation due to both right handed and left handed carpal tunnel release asked me what she could do with her work situation?

> *P. C.:* Now that I am going back to work, what can I do to
> help stay at work? I am on the computer 8 hours a day and

have been at the same job for over fifteen years.

*Grafton:* What is the title of your job?

*P. C:* Administrative Assistant for the City of........

*Grafton:* Did your doctor mention anything about Workers' Compensation?

*P. C:* No, it never came up, I just went to the doctor because my hands hurt and were swollen.

*Grafton:* When you go back to the doctor, ask him to review your medical history, work history, recreation history and ask him what percentage of these hand surgeries are related to your work. Then, take that answer in writing to your Human Resources Director.

*P. C:* What can I do with my workstation to help?

*Grafton:* I have tested you for your dominance and directionality of fingers and hands with your use of the mouse and keypad. So, I recommend moving your mouse to the left hand side, purchasing a left handed mouse and to use the Mouse Training CD as you go back to work at the same job. Also I recommend a telephone ear piece so you can quit holding the phone with your neck while talking.

## WHAT TO DO ABOUT SYMPTOMS
If your medical advisor is recommending surgery as the treatment for your condition of CTS or MSD, according to NIOSH, "such medical (surgery) interventions have met with mixed success, especially when an affected person must return to the same working

conditions."

If you are having trouble with your hands, you can draw a picture of each of your hands and mark the places or your pictures in the areas where you have pain, burning, numbness or swelling. If you believe you have a work-related injury, you need to find out the answers to questions like:

- Can I select what doctor or hospital?
- What benefits will I be entitled to?
- Who is responsible for paying my benefits?
- After treatment, if I am unable to return to my same job, will I be offered retraining?
- Will I be able to receive Social Security Disability benefits as a result of CTS?
- What if my employer fires me or even harasses me about my CTS?

States have their own Workers' Compensation laws. To check on your state, go to their website and you will find what you will be entitled to and what to do if you are having issues with your employer. According to the website search engine, Alta Vista, when I typed in computer related injuries, there were 2,430,000 hits. From the website RSI on Alta Vista "it is not uncommon for people to have to leave computer-dependent careers as a result, or even to be disabled and unable to perform tasks such as driving or dressing themselves" writes Paul Marehausen, a victim in the hazardous occupation of a computer user.

The National Women's Health Information Center recommends to help prevent CTS, take these following precautions. Reduce your force and relax your grip, take frequent breaks, watch your form, improve your posture, keep your hands warm and use ergonomically designed equipment. They also recommend modifying the layouts of workstations and altering the existing method for performing the job task. This is exactly what this book is all about, a new method for performing the task.

For more information about CTS and RSI disease and rehabilitation, refer to the comprehensive book, The Medical Disability Advisor by Presley Reed MD, page 293. If you are having medical problems and you believe your symptoms are suggestive of problems, on your legal pad notes, start a Symptom Checklist you may use to start keeping track of your complaints i.e. when they started, how often and recent dates? Also if you have had treatment for a computer related injury with your hands and it was not deemed workers compensation related, you may wish to investigate if you have disability insurance.

WebMD, from their Actionset/Healthwise setting states to prevent CTS at the keyboard: "Don't wait till you have symptoms to take preventative measures" as measures are well worth the effort. "Increase your awareness of how you use your hands and equipment throughout the day" is their recommendation. Also pay attention to early warnings of trouble.

## SETTING UP A SAFETY PROGRAM

At the 2008 Southeast Voluntary VPPPA convention in Louisville, Ky. speaker John Drebinger encouraged safety-minded professionals to take action with the secret of getting ahead is simply getting started. In his book, Mastering Safety Communication, Drebinger writes you must improve your communication skills for a safe, productive and profitable workplace. I can add, you must have all three to have success in over coming glitches in the fast lane of commuter workstation modifications. If your company is not already a member of this organization, their website is www.vpppa.org. The organization is sponsored by OSHA.

If you are a new human resource person on the job and are encountering numerous complaints and grievances due to computer related injuries, check back with your companies review and analysis of injury and illness records. By this review, you will be able to identify the potential MSD cases with the names given earlier and they may just include ganglion cyst, thoracic outlet syndrome and even entries as hand sprain, wrist sprain, finger tear or even just pain. By looking at each department, division you will be able to pinpoint where the problem is and make your mark within your organization for change.

NIOSH recommends from their prevention article "process redesign is preferable to administrative means such as job rotation. The frequency and severity of CTS can be minimized through training programs that increase worker awareness of symptoms and prevention methods" and of course, the "proper medical management of injured workers."

A good resource of general education series videos may be obtained from your local Arthritis Foundation should your medical advisor recommend this. Carpal tunnel Syndrome, Osteoarthritis, Arthritis on the Job, Diet and Exercise are just some of the names of the videos. Also they have a Medication Series; Aspirin and Other NSAIDS, Corticosteroid Medications, and Methotrexate. With the news of the law suits against the makers of Celebrex and Vioxx, do not be afraid to ask questions of your medical advisor about the use and adverse effects of any of these types of medications.

M. Mani (2000) at the Rollins School of Public Health at Emory University in Atlanta, Georgia in their study of work place injuries stated "Extensive epidemiological investigation indicates that the adverse ergonomic exposures of force, repetition, vibration and certain postures are risk factors for development of many of these disorders. Assessment of patients with possible work-related upper limb disorders requires eliciting information about the illness, performing an examination about the illness, and obtaining information about adverse ergonomic exposures on and off from work." Their conclusions were "Treatment can only be successful when exposure to adverse ergonomic risk factors is reduced or eliminated." With assistance in how you can help set up an Ergonomic program see NIOSH articles from their website.

In the NY Times article on August 12, 2004 by Yingdan Gu, "taking a small step toward redressing that imbalance, a one-handed computer keyboard, the FrogPad, has a new version with lefties in mind." I reviewed the website www.frogpad.com and found "the new keyboard was aimed at both left-handed typists and users of photo-editing and computer-aided-design software." From the FrogPad web site "demand is exploding for a new generation of mobile devices. There is no standard data entry device. For Portability, Miniature keyboards, Thumb Keyboards, Folding keyboards, Electronic Ink, and Voice Recognition are sufficient but not fully functional." "Users are demanding the ability to access and manipulate any data from anywhere at any time" and this "means for users to input and access data." You may wish to review again your checklists and your testing results as you plan on updating your workstation.

"Most office injuries are the result of repetitive actions-typing, using the mouse, 10-key data entry and so on" but "by making just a few minor adjustments in office equipment, you can thwart injuries and sick days" from the Microsoft Small Business Center website. Workers' Compensation costs go down when assessments are completed and training programs instituted. At that same website. "How (can you) put a cap on worker's comp costs" as they "continue to rise and cause pain to more and more small companies." The five suggestions to help in that regard are to "1) Make safety a common goal, not an area of friction. 2) If you've already had claims, institute a better safety program. 3) Don't misrepresent what your employees are doing. 4) Reach out to OSHA. 5) Put some money where your safety mouth is." Investments in safety are training, equipment, instruction and systems. Should you be in a position of authority to review your safety programs and make suggestions, this book has put you on the right road.

## ERGONOMICS

The www.TheErgonomicsCenter.com has initiated a small circular "Datalizer." My interpretation of this guide could easily be used in conjunction with the eTool as the "values were referenced from the 1988 Anthropometric Survey of U. S. Army Personnel." The guide offers a choice of "male only" or "female only."

A Physical Abilities Testing Program was developed by Advanced Ergonomics, Inc. I would recommend jobs requiring six or more hours of computer use, should be included in performance of essential tasks associated with physically demanding jobs. This company uses validation studies, legal defensibility and program effectiveness in their marketing and "is approaching 1,000,000 performed tests for client companies to date in 2008."

The Ergonomics Center of North Carolina asks you to meet "EDGAR." They have developed the "Ergonomic Decision-making Guide for Assessing Risk." This company is there when you need to assess your work areas to identify the risk associated with each of your company's jobs. Most training programs are designed around a step type of process. For example, implementation, IT management, records management and verification requirements. Without management involvement, a training program will not be successful. That is where corporate America can be the rise or fall of ergonomics as we know it. The costs of worker injuries must be compared with the costs of ergonomics.

One such Best Practice presentation by Barb Tate and Charles Moore from the Monsanto, Augusta, Georgia Plant outlined their training management as a Four Step Process into a Modular Training Program. These program design objectives are comprehensive ensuring all department personnel receive sufficient training to perform their job functions which require systematic documentation, demonstration of acquired knowledge/skills via written tests and interviews within their paperless computer programs.

In the Ergonomists's Corner newsletter, Jim Briggs, OTR/L asks why your company should offer worksite wellness programs. In addition to reducing Workers' Comp/Disability and reducing injuries, many potential problems can be corrected by worksite modification, employee wellness programs and retraining. His statement "ergonomic interventions" are worth the costs. Briggs recommends staging: storage and positioning of materials, supplies, location of the work area and the availability of equipment. Briggs concludes ergonomic interventions are not foolproof and the employee may need to be assessed against the physical demands of the job. Another tip in the newsletter, "the body wants and needs to change during the day and should include mousing or reading from the screen."

Megan Youngblood asks "Is your office a petri dish? Many companies have 24/7 computer data employees: banks, healthcare. These employees share computers and workstations. Youngblood states the prime habitats for the viruses that cause colds and flu are desks, phones and computer keyboards. Actually any transfer point would be the touch points of these habitats. These were important issues raised from this article's January 2008 in the Magazine of NW Florida's Business section.

Dr. Charles P. Gerba, a microbiologist from the University of Arizona, and the Clorox Company, tested phones, desks and computer mice within a variety of different occupations. They discovered the most bacteria per inch were found on surfaces used by school teachers because of their constant contact with children. Accountants ranked second to teachers, followed by bankers, radio disc jockeys and doctors. Even the smallest traces of bacteria were found in the offices of consultants, publicists and lawyers.

Several studies recommend keeping a hand sanitizer with alcohol concentration above 60 percent to be effective. Purell and Clean-Well are two products listed as hand sanitizers and disinfectant wipes.

NASA's 1970's study by Bill Wolverton, Ph.D., had concerns for office safety which included air quality. They recommended surround your office space with low-maintenance houseplants like snake, spider, ivy and/or ficus plants. Common houseplants have the ability to reduce carbon dioxide and vapors from toxic, irritating volatile organic compounds.

Check to see if your company has or uses a Physical Abilities Test for new hires or employees returning to work after an injury. If your company does use this type of test, find out if a validation study was performed. If a validation test was not done, your company would not be able to defend against a discrimination complaint. Also check to see if the validation requirements fit into the CFR-20 Chapter 60–3 US Department of Labor. The validation test must be based on a thorough job analysis and not just on a job description, normative data or a reference such as the Dictionary of Occupational Titles, a job task analysis and/or statements from the employer saying the test is representative of the job is not a qualified validation document. Another item to check is whether the validation document has an analysis of adverse impact. Their pass rates are different for male and females and those over forty. If you are caught in the throws of an OFCCP audit or EEOC challenge, the agency will ask for the validation study and the adverse impact analysis. Now that you are interested in this top of validation, check to see if the vendor periodically reviews the requirements as it is an on-going process. Physical Abilities Testing programs that are well-designed can reduce injuries by 20% to 50%. By knowing these procedures, you will be a step up in eliminating a large part of your workers compensation injuries before they happen with better employee selection.

Custom training solutions by professional trainers appears to be common-place for corporate America. If you give your employees the tools they need to grow, you can watch your business grow too. By building teamwork within the office you can increase productivity, generate creative solutions, uncover employee talents and tap into a common mission. With the development of ownership mentality there are limitless possibilities to improve employee retention, uncover employee talents just by discovering new work tools.

According to the Employee Law Guide published by the U. S. Dept. of Labor, you have "the right to complain to OSHA about safety and health conditions in their workplaces and, to the extent permitted by law, have their identities kept confidential from employers, contest the amount of time OSHA allows for correcting violations of standards, and participate in OSHA workplace inspections." If you need any type of training and education assistance, contact one of the field offices for technical advice in your state. OSHA's toll free number is 1-800-321-6742.

At the website Kids Health "only a small percentage of kids have RSI. You can help prevent RSI by taking preventive measures and redesigning your home computer environment so that it fits your child." "Taking frequent breaks is also an important step in preventing repetitive stress injuries. Your child may lose track of time and forget to take breaks, so it's your job to make sure she rests her eyes, back, wrists, and neck every half hour or so."

I believe that Information Technology (IT) managers and their departments are a very important part of the process that needs to be educated and informed in order to decrease this trend in cost and statistics. Not only are they the ones purchasing the equipment they are also involved in setting up the initial workplace. This epidemic has just as much impact on the employer as it does on the employee. No amount of ergonomic changes, fancy keyboards, or exercises is going to help if you are simply typing more than your body can handle. Don't try to be the fastest, most powerful hacker around — the cost is too high. Also, is there recreational computer use you can reduce? Can some of your electronic mail messages be replaced by telephone calls or conversations in person? And lose the computer/video games... which often involve long, unbroken sessions of *very* tense keyboard or controller use. If nothing else, pause the game every 3–4 minutes. Don't sacrifice your hands to a game!

There is a dollar amount that can be put into an ergonomics program. Productivity increases and performance improves when employees keep their minds on their work and aren't concerned about pain or the difficulty of the job. What is especially difficult to grasp is the concrete dollar value of benefits and productivity in the white-collar computer environment. A question may be asked am I getting my money's worth. One comment was "Our ergonomics program bought everyone new wrist rests, but I approved the purchase just to shut everyone up. I think it's just a bunch of baloney," says another. What will it cost is the usual question raised by another. I sure don't see any direct impact on my bottom line is the usual comment from a skeptic manager. Fixing a workstation averages $150 per year. Employers will pay $4.2 billion (including $875 million now lost by workers whose income and benefits are not fully covered by workers' compensation).

White-collar industries such as insurance companies have shown improvements by ergonomic interventions in worker performance and productivity. Improvements are illustrated by tracking such things as hours worked, units processed, quality audits made, number of analyst contracts, and amount of processable work activity. Ergonomic interventions in the workstations can be shown to impact these areas directly if baselines are established before and after interventions. A key is to track productivity according to client methodology; then improvements can become clear. If tasks can be assigned a value and time/benefit ratio, they can be compared to management goals and can easily be tracked for dollar significance.

The basic idea is teaming with a senior-level manager to determine the best way to measure ergonomic interventions. What many ergonomists fail to understand is that first of all, an all-important baseline is needed to measure against. This baseline shows where the organization is in terms of throughput. It shows how the organization is working now, before ergonomic changes. This measurement must be taken prior to intervention so improvements can be properly charted. Before making any modifications to workflow, methods, or workstations, you must have something to measure against — generally, the current level of productivity.

I must reinforce to you computer related injuries is a world-wide issue. The Australian Disability organization has general suggestions to reduce other ways to reduce the risk of computer related injuries include: Make sure your work space is well ventilated. Maintain equipment, such as laser printers and photocopiers, to reduce emissions.

In his article that is useful for a Best Practice training program is to focus on models according to the website www.ecsu.edu . Ray Fleming recommends seeking a Policy Analyst for your ergonomics program. Fleming states many Policy Analysts rely upon models with diminishing marginal benefits and increasing marginal costs for pollution prevention past a certain threshold of quality. While this model is valid and useful in many instances, applying it to the present health risks is problematic for several reasons. Fleming acknowledges that "first, each individual has a different threshold of pain, so it is difficult to generalize about acceptable pain levels across a population" especially if the injured worker is working with pain. Secondly, Fleming explains "while an individual could use this model on a personal basis, the relationship between tissue damage, pain, and loss of function is not well understood," nor is it likely to be a simple function. After a claim has been filed for a computer related injury, "the recovery times are often much longer than the injury times, particularly during recovery from acute injury." The challenge according to Fleming is managing the health risks as they can be complicated. These types of cases are complicated by the associated social risk landscape. The social impacts are even more variable and difficult to quantify, but they are nonetheless present.

The social risks are less well documented and are often unapparent to non-injured parties. Fleming concludes by saying "for young professionals and college students accustomed to using the computer as an integrated part of their life and work, the social losses incurred through computer non-usage can be quite high."

NIOSH/NORA is working with safety training products. NIOSH evaluates training effectiveness by using audience surveys, focus groups, computer-based laboratory testing, field studies, statistical analyses, education and curriculum development and development of training materials from brochures to videos.

In 2007, a NORA project was begun to investigate a "Work Organization Intervention in IRS Service Centers" by Paula Grubb, Ph.D. The scope of the project will assess the success of an intervention to improve the work climate, employee satisfaction, health, and well-being and suggest preventive measures to discover personnel stress levels. NIOSH will work with the National Treasury Employees Union in making recommendations for refining and further implementing the enhanced supervisory practices intervention model.

In this last section on ergonomics, safety and types of programs that are in place, we will agree that the best definition in ergonomics is fitting the task to the human based on their dominance. But what can you personally do to help? The association of physical factors and personal factors are multifactorial according to the plastic surgeon Karpitskay Y. (2002).

There results support the reports that factors as obesity, hypothyroidism and diabetes were very prevalent in their case control study. So, lifestyle change and good medical care can reduce your factors for risk for Carpal Tunnel Syndrome. Know what your risk factors are.

You can help prevent problems by diet, check your body weight frequently, exercise and are you taking glucosamine? The OTC medications are so controversial. If you have swelling of your hand or fingers, for the short term use rest, ice, compression and elevation (RICE). But, for the long term, see your medical advisor. And of course, as you turn on your computer for the day, do your hand, finger, arm and upper body warm ups. Continue to make yourself responsible for your computer health at your workstation.

# CHAPTER TWENTY

*Legends of prediction are common throughout the whole Household of Man. Gods speak, spirits speak, and computers speak. Oracular ambiguity or statistical probability provides loopholes, and discrepancies are expunged by Faith.*

**Ursula K. LeGuin**

## WHEN LEFT IS RIGHT

At the time of this writing I am still reviewing daily the development of various input devices as explained in my idea of the dual numerical keyboard and other office machines with numerical changes as this book suggests with patent development. I am also following closely the new products from the electronic stores and their web sites daily. Just as I must follow that closely, I also must follow the politics behind all of the ergonomics associated with CTS, RSI et al.

I truly believed in November 1999, after ten years of research, discussion and compromise, (President Clinton signed into law the Ergonomic Standards), that more would be done for the American worker. Two months later, President Bush signed legislation repealing the Ergonomic Standards. Since the repeal over 500,000 American Workers have suffered unnecessarily according to the AFL-CIO website. If you work for the Dept. of Defense, you can view their website www.aflcio.org and view their recommendations for safety. Every 18 seconds an American worker gets an MSD. I agree with their statement, you must "work with management to improve your work station." But you need to be armed with the information

219

found in this book to support that effort.

## EXPECTATIONS AND LESSONS LEARNED

I hope you can see why I recommended for keypad data entry training to focus on speed, pacing and rhythm of the non preferred left hand and also to determine if you are a verbal or visual learner. You learned a technique for relaxation training (deep breathing, visual imaging), completing finger movements with the eyes closed, eyes closed and the beat to music, eyes closed and alternating hands/finger movements. By keeping the eyes open in practicing finger movements will allow the right brain to encode a picture of this image.

I hope you had fun with the coordination experiments. Did I provoke your thinking about yourself and the how and why you do things the way you do with the Blau Torque test and Wilke-Sheeley finger circling test?

When I made the statement the computer and the computer user appear to be 'one' instigated more research about computers and software and I hope you will continue to keep your mind and your eyes open to new technology.

In 1982 the computer was named "Man of the Year" by Time Magazine. Hardware and software makers focus on enhancing your PC's or laptop performance. With the millions of dollars spent on patents and research and development projects within computer companies, why in the world did these companies not focus more on human capabilities with the use of hands and fingers first before moving computers to the market? The Romans put the cart before the horse. Railroad Engineers put the cars before the tracks. Why not put the human body into the further development of computer operating systems. If computer companies do not have human motor learning specialists within their job descriptions, I recommend they work with OSHA to develop this within their Best Practice methods.

## TECHNIQUES TO ENHANCE TRAINING
- My plan for you as you worked through the chapters was to:
- Expand your knowledge of computer related overuse injuries.
- Recognize the muscles and tendons of the hand.
- Gain knowledge of brain organization to assist in understanding coordination of the extremities.
- Identify the types of treatment and diagnosis for hand injuries.
- Recognize occupational titles at risk for CTS, RSI and MSD.
- Know the types of dominance. and preferences in the hands and fingers.
- Know the steps for training and education of the non preferred left hand.
- Understand input devices/products needed for dual systems.
- Use the assessment checklists available from OSHA, NIOSH and BLS to examine your work station.
- Know the types of exercises used for warm up, rest or for stretching for the hands, fingers, shoulders, arms and back.
- Have the ability to assess mirror image or parallel directionality between the hands and fingers.
- Know how to institute a training program at work.

You also learned where to purchase or availability of stand alone numeric keypads, either right to left pattern sequence or left to right pattern sequence or keyboards with either right to left pattern sequence or left to right pattern on the left side of the computer keyboard With learning the patterns of finger movements you will understand why your little finger and the other fingers differ in their ease of movement together. These recommendations include decisions about where you should have your mouse at your workstation and of course what type to buy.

For more training tips, add the metronome, then add music for rhythm training. You probably did not understand why I included the research on musicians, so now you know. Also I recommend morning training, daily 5x a week, (14) 50 minute sessions with a 10 minute break in between each session and adequate rest between sessions. If you did not find keyboard labels for letters or numbers, you can purchase Giant Keyboard Labels for $2.99 from the Miles Kimball catalog, www.mileskimball.com or from piengineering. com, the labels come with the keypad.

On site work site training is recommended. If you have not already discussed this book with your Human Resources Manager, now may be a good time. If you are in the vocational education training and retraining profession, you may wish to show this book to the employer. A training suggestion for HR staff are to add 1) elements of competency and performance criteria, 2) data entered using relevant equipment according to policy and procedure, and 3) data entered and within designated time limits.

Of course, if you work for yourself at home, it may be easier to get this training started. But, I will add a bit of information at the end of this chapter about jobs and if your supervisor needs help in establishing an ergonomic program at work using NIOSH guidelines found on the web. You will be more than armed with information for you and your fellow employees.

Variables include 1) practices, 2) knowledge, and 3) requirements. Large companies have Risk Management Departments that have developed Return to Work programs. These programs have Transitional Duty and Light Duty Jobs. By having these jobs, employers can expect to reduce workers compensation claim costs by an average of 30 percent by establishing and maintaining a Return to Work Program.

Boller in his book What Color is Your Parachute? captured perspectives on creativity and the brain. Constant are new findings in knowing more about the brain that it is difficult to "keep up." While our whole educational system is oriented toward people with verbal skills rather than intuitive: toward achievement (performance) rather than relationship, goals will change through education.

My expectations have been, performance will be greater in women workers, left handers will have greater performance than right handers, strong right handers tend to move both left and right index fingers in the opposite directions and familial left handers tend to move both left and right index fingers in the same directions. Did you find your expectations similar to those mentioned above? If you have not already done so, check with your family history of left handedness (sinistrals) and sinistral family members as they are more bilateralized. In other words, are they mixed handers or ambidextrous in their handedness?

Congratulations in selecting your electronic devices and completing this series of steps in learning how to use your non preferred hand and ready to reduce the number of repetitions from your right hand and move some of them to the left hand and fingers. To maintain your excellence, practice, practice, practice. Look at it as a game. In many instances of computer games for children and/or adults, use of both hands are paramount. This will help your use of the left hand. Richard Restak, Neurologist and writer, states "practice your chosen manual skill enough to establish and maintain the brain circuits devoted to that skill." I hope your goals are the same as mine and Dr. Restak's "to establish and enhance your brain's performance by maintaining your manual skill levels in an area of your own choosing."

In a discussion about directionality of the non preferred hand with Mathew Monroe, computer programmer with a computer games development company (Liquid Light, LLC), we found we had similar interests in how to deal with the left hand learning. Most computer games require use of both hands, and as the programs are written, you must keep in mind how the hands work. Monroe explained programming and software development takes both hands used in unison to be successful. There is a tremendous amount of typing involved using both hands continuously. Working with the graphics part of developing there is a strong usage of the dominant hand because of the precision needed from the mouse (to draw images and shade).

Monroe continued stating mirroring is the most common way he has seen in the work place. Many of the people he has worked with their weak (left) hand have found the tasks are much easier to learn on a mirrored keyboard. Monroe believes the ability to switch hands and remain effective would be a huge asset in the workplace. Monroe first became interested in how the hands work at an early age, around 15 or 16. He was very interested in sports at school and knew ambidexterity in sports was a plus. So, he started training himself to use his left hand, which was the weak hand. Then he learned how he was 'mirrored' in the way his left hand responded to his right. If he thought about dribbling the basketball with his left hand, he found it was easier to do the opposite of the way he would do it with his right hand.

If you think about sports skills as they relate to computer keyboard workstation skills, they are very similar. It is a plus in baseball or softball to be mixed handed or ambidextrous as well as basketball, tennis, fencing or hockey.

So why not develop the idea to be a Computer Jock or a Computer Jill. You can set up your workstation with both numerical keypad and mouse and have a dual set up. As you review all of your checklists and your notes, I believe you will be surprised at the elements to consider in setting up your revised workstation. While you are waiting for your computer to download, do the hand, finger and upper arm exercises for your warm-up.

From eMarketerDaily.com, June 24, 2005 issue, by 2010, over 54 million households will own one video game console and most will have a portable system and a non-portable system. More than half the households in the United States have a computer so computer use will only escalate within the home and for most of you, your work life too. Computer use is in. So, protect your hands and fingers. I would anticipate that many changes will be made in the computer keyboards due to overuse injuries. With the new iPhones, text messaging with PDAs, new types of treatments will need to found or invented.

Be sure and remember your relaxation techniques. It has been shown in EMG studies the upper back and neck muscles become tight. Learn how to relax those specific muscles too. If you have use of the Internet with your computer, go to http://www.osha.gov/SLTC/etools/computerworkstations/components_keyboards.html and you will see how the U. S. Department of Labor recommends Computer Workstations. This department recognizes the need for monitoring due to the large number of computer related injuries. Their recommendations ask you to consider your keyboard placement (height and distance), design and use and left hand key usage. Their instructions point out potential hazards, possible solutions. For left hand key usage programmable stand alone keypads are available which can be programmed to facilitate either right or left hand usage.

At the website www.highbeam.com/library my query for motor control, training, computer and overuse injuries states Area Ergonomics Specialists Emphasize Injury Prevention. If you are still using the mouse on the right side of the computer and you wish to move the mouse to the left side of the computer, use the same directionality exercises to determine which mouse to select as they are made with clickers on both sides. You can also program your mouse on your computer by going to Control Panel, Hardware, then Mouse, then, Button Configuration.

Office workers do not endure the physical riggers of laying concrete, fighting fires like those of other occupations. But, repetitive activities such as computer usage, their bodies may see a fair share of ache and wear. Melvin Saunders at www.braincourse.com states to be able to use both hands equally well, practice is the key. Saunders appears to be well versed in the ways to train yourself to be ambidextrous. Ancient history shows ambidexterity was promoted but just by looking at standard keyboards that is not the case. Saunders recommends "wherever you would use your one hand, use the other instead — putting a key in the door, combing your hair, brushing your teeth" just pay attention and use your left hand more by "consciously switching when you are about ready to do something", like pouring a glass of water or tea. My statement Left is Right at the beginning is based on two facts. The first, it is a right handers world. Second, in the case of computers, being left hand dominant will make it easier to use the left side computer devices to reduce the load on the computer keyboard and keypad system.

## BIAS IN THE WORKPLACE

Earlier in the book I asked the question, is their discrimination against left handers in general. Yes, there is. But, it a matter of human function. The issue of left handedness can be found in education, sports and even in medicine. Left handedness will continue to be researched as there are so many peculiarities in left handers. In Europe and the Asian nations, left handedness is less than 2%, so there is definitely discrimination there.

That brings up a question raised by M. Siebner. (2002) asking if there are "Long Term consequences of switching handedness:" "A positron emission tomography study on handwriting in 'converted' left handers" was completed in the Institute of Neurology in London. Many left handers in other countries, especially "German schools forced" their students "to learn to write with their right hand." Their "findings provide evidence for persisting differences in the functional neuroanatomy of handwriting between right handers and converted left handers, despite decades of right hand writing." So, it looks as if once a left hander, always a left hander in the primary sensorimotor cortex of the brain. With this method of training, pay close attention to mixed handers and the computer user's nationality.

In an Interview with Jan, an English teacher in Ft. Worth, Texas:

*Grafton:* You have read my book, so my question is when you were working in the lab what did you do for the left handers in the class?

*Jan:* When I was in the Computer Lab, the only thing we could do for "lefties" was to change the side of the keyboard the mouse was plugged into. Because of an injury (not computer related) to my right hand years ago, I was forced to "learn" how to perform many tasks with my left hand. This actually helped me a lot, and I still practice using my left hand. I do not consider myself ambidextrous because of that, but I do not feel like I over burden my right hand any longer.

## LAPTOPS AND WIRELESS HANDHELDS

Laptops Now More Popular Than Desktops is the headline on June 4, 2005 from the San Francisco Newswire. The price drop and quality have improved and the computing crowd is increasingly requiring mobility. Last year, 80% of notebooks offered wireless but this has increased by 15%. In 2005, more laptops were sold than desk top models. Doctors have warned for years that repeated thumb use on laptops and video game controllers can cause osteoarthritis. Thumb problems will continue according to Sean Hughes of the Imperial College of London told the BBC that excessive text-messaging and use of the BlackBerry wireless communications device can be harmful to users. The thumb is designed to flex and rotate in all directions and works differently from other fingers. Alen Hedge, from Cornell University, told UPI, thumb injuries are not new. When video gaming came in, then washer woman's thumb became known as Nintendo thumb and now it is referred to as Blackberry Thumb.

From The Yankee Group research organization, "estimates are there will be 60 million wireless data devices in the United States by 2005." Cahners In-Stat/MDR "predicts that by 2005, more than

50% of 900 million cellular phones sold will be data enabled." Over two weeks ago, a new cellular phone with the mirrored numerical keypad was shown in an announcement. The race is on to see who or what company can develop the best numerical pads that are productive whether it is wireless or a plug in.

If you are already disabled with your hands and arms, a new government program is available if you are interested in telephonic and electronic (computer) programs. The program is entitled CAPS Training. The web site is www.tricare.osd.mil/cap. This was announced July 8, 2004 by Labor Secretary Chao.

Do not become a workers' compensation statistic. Put this book's information in your hands and train both hands for data management. Or if you are in the professional medical field, use this information to reduce workplace injuries. In today's world, to grow professionally means learning new skills. Since technology changes so frequently, the new skill from last year may become obsolete in a year's time. You must continuously secure your job and enhance your employability even at the same job you hold.

Finally, "workers who use computers earn more than those who do not." The Bureau of Labor states "we find that long-run returns to computer use are over 5% for most workers." So, it will behoove you to make all efforts to equalize your work station and work habits to use your dominance to your best advantage. What I hope within ten years is to see dual keyboards in your computer learning at your high school or middle school that are individualized and then you take them with you. You will know early where you should place your mouse. Education is the key for reduction in work injuries. Pay close attention to what our government is recommending for ergonomic improvements at your work station.

The Department of Commerce issued a statement in June 2005 estimating internet users in the United States was up for broadband users 105.1 million and dial up closely behind at 70.3 million users. So, there are a lot of computer keyboarders that need the information in this book.

The Bibliography section is there for you to follow up on any of the studies mentioned and how to find it in your university library system or for the books, in your local library. Generic equipment seems to be the standard of the large computer and keyboard with software development. But, due to computer related work injuries, non generic equipment has been developed by the smaller companies' world wide. In marketing studies of computers and the workstation, you are not limited in what you can use. For example, in golf, you are limited to 14 clubs in the bag. If you decided on a dual system of both numeric keypads and/or mouse addition, there is nothing wrong with that.

Accountants, Programmers, Writers and CAD workers will enjoy what this book has to offer them. So, I hope you have paid attention to the OSHA checklists, NIOSH, all the devices available, training method for the left hand for numerical keypad and mouse to make the correct decision where you are heading to prevent or further prevent any upper extremity injury. And do not forget; add the exercises as you start your computer day.

The secret of keyboarding for success is practice. Does practice make perfect? No, practice makes permanent. A permanent imprint by network development within your brain. Good luck in your computing using your left hand and fingers for numerical data entry or mouse changes. Walter Elliott is quoted stating Perseverance is not a long race; it is many short races one after another! If you know someone who needs this book, give a helping hand. Help someone by passing the book on.

# FREQUENTLY ASKED QUESTIONS

**Question**

I am a right handed female office worker. Will it be easier for me to learn the left hand use system than my male counterparts in this office?

**Answer**

According to the Cortex article in 2001 by Nalcaci, "Results confirmed that right handed females tend to have more asymmetric motor function than right handed males."

---

**Question**

Are workers who develop Carpal Tunnel Syndrome (CTS) or other types of Repetitive Stress injuries (RSI) protected by the Americans with Disabilities Act?

**Answer**

Computers and keyboards require a safety guideline such as "warning." Also, courts have ruled that in situations where CTS and RSI progress to the state in which they are considered "serious and permanent" (some degree of nerve damage, surgery), they qualify as "disabilities" under the ADA. One of the protections afforded workers with CTS under the ADA requires employers to provide them with a "reasonable accommodation" to allow them to perform the basic functions of their job.

**Question**

Explain ADA and type of accommodation.

**Answer**

An employer of a computer operator with CTS might be required to accommodate the worker with: An ergonomically modified workstation; Reduction in computer work from 8 hours to 4 or 5 hours per day, allowing the worker to perform non-computer related tasks for a portion of the day; Voice activated software; And if qualified, transfer the computer operator to a different job within the company, which does not require computer work. By denying a "reasonable accommodation" to a worker with CTS, the employer will be deemed to have engaged in prohibited discrimination under the ADA. CAP accommodates our Federal-partnered employees with disabilities who telework as a form of reasonable accommodation."

---

**Question**

I bought a left handed keyboard/keypad as I was having problems with my right hand but it is just too hard for me to do without looking at the keypad numbers. Can you help?

**Answer**

First, you did not say if the keypad numbers on the left side went left to right or right to left. I suspect the numbers are going left to right. You probably need right to left. That is explained using Dr. Blau's book about his Torque Test. Also the Temprado study in 2005 concluded the "results suggest that learning and transfer of coordination patterns is mediated by abstract directional codes that become part of the memory.

---

**Question**

I write with my left hand but I play sports like tennis with my right hand. I am in college trying to learn to be an accountant but I am having trouble learning the keypad numbers without looking. Is there anything I can do?

**Answer**

"Handedness is not a one- dimensional trait or behavior" according to Corey (2001) in the Neuropsychiatry/Neuropsychology Behavior Journal. These researchers at Tulane University believe multiple measures that assess different aspects of hand preference and performance" should be used and mention there are "implications for hemispheric specialization." Review the summary by Wilke and Sheeley in my book as that explains the difference between the hands and the fingers in directionality. I recommend for you to review closely the picture of the dual keyboard and keypad and go over the numbers on the keypad with your hands and fingers and figure out by your hand's touch what type of keypad you should use for either the right hand or the left hand.

---

**Question**

I am trying out the system of the dual keypad but I am so much slower using my left hand, why?

**Answer**

My answer refers to the study by Fearing in 2001 at Tulane University who indicate in their studies of right handers and left handers without verbal prompting or interference found "that individuals with a stronger right hand preference tended to tap at a higher rate on the right side." Try out some of my suggestions for help learning left hand usage.

---

**Question**

My brother and I are twins. I am right handed, he is left handed. We have taken your Torque Test and we are not the same at all. Can you explain?

**Answer**

Look at the graph by Dr. Blau showing 8 different torque examples.

In the study by Mathey in 1979, he suggests "there is a genetic influence" in "circling patterns."

---

**Question**

I am a new bookkeeper on my first job. I am right handed. I have been looking at your suggestions but I am not sure about what I should concentrate on when using the keypad and inputting numbers. Do you have other suggestions?

**Answer**

In a study by Woods in 1980, they looked at "Torque, hemispheric dominance and psychosocial adjustment" in "Concurrent Counting and Typing: Lateralized Interference depends on a difference between the hands in a motor skill." When you are doing two tasks at one time (dual performance), there can be interference in processing. What I recommend is to learn to focus on the numbers, not counting at the same time. If you were a left hander, then their study indicates, left handers can do both (counting and typing) at the same time.

---

**Question**

We took your suggestions as a family exploration since we all use computers. After we took the Torque Test, all of my children show different types of torque. Can you explain?

**Answer**

From a study by Scheirs in 1990 found in Neuropsycholgia Journal, " Relationship between the direction of movements and handedness in children "and "circling, for instance, was predominantly clockwise in the youngest and counter-clockwise in the older children." So, it would seem that to interpret that finding, experience in use of the hands could change depending upon the type of manual tasks you do.

---

**Question**

I am right handed, female, and I really want to learn the dual system of keyboards. Will it help to use the rubber band exercises on my left hand to help this learning?

**Answer**

In the Farthing study in 2005 in the journal Medicine and Science Sports Exercise, this group of researchers found "cross education with hand strength training occurs only in the right to left direction of transfer in right handed individuals.. We conclude that cross education of arm muscular strength is most pronounced to the non dominant arm."

I can only conclude, yes, it will help.

---

**Question**

My job requires me to be on the computer 8–10 hours daily. Both of my arms and hands get tired, especially my left hand. I am a right handed, female.

**Answer**

In the European Journal of Applied Physiology and Occupational Physiology study by Yasuda in1983, they found from their "results it is suggested that increase of blood flow in the contralateral limb after training may, at least in part, be related to the cross transfer effect of muscular endurance." I recommend both warm-up and rest break exercise regimen for you to include the hand strength ball exercise for both hands and arms.

---

**Question**

My job as a research librarian requires me to not only use my computer but to monitor and assist 12 other students with their research on the computer. I am left handed and I am having tendonitis in my right arm and index finger?

**Answer**

Be sure and review the exercise regimen information, then add the warm-up and rest break exercises to your desk top. Also on your computer in your office and at home, obtain a wireless mouse and use your left hand as much as possible. Also review two websites: Fentek Industries for alternative input devices and tifac.com to become very educated how this problem occurred while working.

---

**Question**

Will your hand and finger exercises really help me by strengthening both of my hands? I work 12 hour shifts 3–4 days per week and I am a right handed female.

**Answer**

Yes, from the research as above and this study by Hortobagyi 1997 at East Carolina University by their Biomechanics Laboratory researchers. From the journal Medicine and Science Sports Exercise, page 107, entitled "Greater cross education following training with muscle lengthening than shortening" they concluded using biceps training, "the greater cross education following training was most likely being mediated by both afferent and efferent mechanisms that allow previously sedentary subjects to achieve a greater activation of the untrained limb musculature." In other words, lay your arm down on the workstation table, straighten your arm, and squeeze the ball. Strengthen both arms.

---

**Question**

My wrists hurt when I type, will an alternately designed keyboard help?

**Answer**

It could but the deciding factor is what is causing the wrists to be in pain when you type. An alternately designed keyboard will improve your wrist posture. If this is the primary risk factor causing you pain then the keyboard will reduce or eliminating the pain you are experiencing. However there are other risk factors associated with typing they are repetition (strokes per minute) duration (how long do you type during the day), work rest scheduling (do you take small frequent breaks 1–5 minutes during the day), force used to strike the keys, and contact stress (are the wrists resting on a hard or sharp surface when typing or are you wearing tight fitting jewelry such as a watch or bracelet on the wrist. A new keyboard may help but it is important to examine the other risk factors you are exposed to. This is advice from the Dept. of Defense Ergonomic News

**Question**
Why does my shoulder hurt when I use my mouse?

**Answer**
Many workstations were designed and purchased before the advent of mouse driven software. Think back 10 years ago, if you wanted to use your file manager you hit shift and the F7 keys or spell check was Ctrl and F2. Now to do virtually any command you use a mouse. Workstations that are designed for mouse driven software have an adjustable tray that moves up and down and is large enough to accommodate a keyboard, wrist rest and mouse. My guess is your workstation does not have a keyboard tray that can fit all the above-mentioned items. Since not using a mouse is not an option your mouse rests on top of your desk, whenever you use your mouse you must fully extend your arm. This full arm extension causes stress to the shoulder since the shoulder muscle now must support the entire weight of your arm. As a rule of thumb the elbows should be bent 90 degrees and be close to your sides whenever you type or mouse.

**Question**
What safety guidelines should I follow when using my laptop computer?

**Answer**
The ideal ergonomic computer workstation includes an adjustable desk and chair with a separate computer screen, keyboard, and mouse. Adjustable furniture and separate computer components can be made to *fit* your needs, rather than you trying to adjust to the limitations of the workstation.

But the design of laptop computers defies these basic ergonomic guidelines. Laptop users set up shop on any available surface, often in cramped spaces — a classroom desk, a conference table, an airplane tray, a hotel bed, and their own laps. Chairs are anything available to sit on from a folding chair to a lobby couch to a park bench. The computer screen, keyboard, and mouse are all-in-one units that create a single, fixed design with typically smaller features than in a standard computer set-up.

---

### WHERE CAN I FIND MORE INFORMATION?
Creating the Ideal Computer Workstation: A Step-by-Step Guide, it can be found on the internet at http://chppm-www.apgea.mil/ergowg2/index.htm

# BIBLIOGRAPHY

## STUDIES

Ackland, T., & Hendrie, G., Training the non-preferred hand for fine motor control using a computer mouse, <u>School of Human Movement and Exercise Science</u>, The University of Western Australia, 35 Stirling Hwy, Crawley, WA 600.

Andree M. & Maitra K. Intermanual transfer of a new writing occupation in young adults without disability. <u>Occup. Ther. Int.</u>, 2002, 9 (1):41–56.

Armstrong T., Foulke J., Martin B., Gerson J., & Rempel D. Investigation of applied forces in alphanumeric keyboard work. <u>Center for Ergonomics</u>, University of Michigan, Ann Arbor 48108-2177.

Australia Alexander, Melody, W, & Arp, L., Teaching Ergonomic Techniques: Practices and Perceptions of Secondary Postsecondary Business Educators. <u>CIJE</u>; (1997-00-00) EJ551563.

Amunts K., Jancke L., Mohlberg H., & Steinmetz, K. Interhemispheric asymmetry of the human motor cortex related to handedness and gener. <u>Neuropsychologia</u>. 2000, 38 (3):304–12.

Annett M. & Alexander M. Atypical cerebral dominance: predictions and tests of the right shift theory. <u>Neuropsychologia</u>, 1996 Dec; 34 (12):1215–27.

Appleton, Wis.-Area Ergonomics Specialists Emphasize Injury Prevention, Knight Ridder/Tribune Business News; 5/22/02.

Atcheson, S., Ward, J., & Wing L. <u>Archives of Internal Medicine</u>, Vol. 158 No. 14, July 27, 1998.158:1506–1512.

Bandler, R. & Grinder J. <u>The Structure of Magic</u>, Vol. 1. 1975. Science and Behavior Books, Palo Alto, Calif.

Banks, M., Ghose, T., & Hillis J. Atypical cerebral dominance: predictions and tests of the right shift theory. <u>Vision Res</u>. 2004, Feb. 44 (3) 229–34.

Beredjiklian, P., Bozentka, D., Steinberg, D., & Bernstein J. Evaluating the source and content of orthopaedic information on the Internet. The case of carpal tunnel syndrome. <u>Journal Bone Joint Surg. Am.</u> 2000, Nov. 82-A (11):1540–3.

Blankenburg, F., Ruben, J., Meyer R., Schwiemann J., & Villringer A. Evidence for a rostra-to-caudal somatoptopic organization in human primary somatosensory cortex with mirror-reversal in areas 3b and 1. <u>Cereb. Cortex</u>. 2003, Sep.13 (9): 987–93.

Boadella, J., Sluiter J., & Frings-Dresin M., Reliability of upper extremity tests measured the Ergoas work simulator: a pilot study, <u>Journal Occup. Rehabil.</u> 2003, Dec.13 (4):219–32.

Braun, C., Hess, H., Burkhardt, M., Wuhle, A., & Preissl, H. The Right hand knows what the left hand is feeling. Exp. Brain Res. 2005 Apr. (16293):366–73 Epub 2004 Dec. 10.

Byl, N., & McKenzie, A. Treatment effectiveness for patients with a history of repetitive hand use and focal hand dystonia: a planned, prospective follow-up study. J. Hand Ther. 2000, Oct-Dec.13 (4):289–301.

Cail, F., & Aptel, M. Biomechanical stresses in computer aided design and in data entry. Int. J. Occup. Saf. Ergon. 2003. 9 (3):235–55.

Carson, R., Thomas, J., Summers, J., Walter, M., & Semjen, A. The dynamics of bimanual circle drawing. Q. J. Exp. Psychol. A. 1997, Aug.50 (3):664–83.

Cattaert, D., Semjen, A., & Summers, J. Simulating a neural cross talk model for between hand interference during bimanual circle drawing. Biol. Cybern. 1999 Oct; 81 (4):343–58.

Cheyne, D., Weinberg, H, Gaetz, W., & Jantzen, K. Motor cortex activity and predicting side of movement: neural network and dipole analysis of pre-movement magnetic fields. Neuroscience. Letters. 1995 Mar 24; 188 (2):81–4.

Clancy, Maureen. Children and Safe Computing: Keeping Your Child RSI-Free. (1999-06-00) ED433129.

Computing News, How to Design Your Data Entry for Transfer into SAS or SPSS: the Excel Advantage, robinh@uoregon.edu.

Cramer, S., Finklestein, S., Schaechter, J., Bush, G., & Rosen, B. Activation of distinct motor cortex regions during ipsilateral and contralateral finger movements. J. Neurophysiol. 1999, Jan.8 1 (1):383–7.

Cue, S., Li, E., Zang, Y., Weng, X., Ivry, R., & Wang, J. Both sides of human cerebellum involved in preparation and execution of sequential movements. Neuroreport. 2000, Nov 27; 11 (17):3849–53.

Delisle, A., Imbeau, D., Santos, B., Plamondon, A., & Montpetit, Y. Left-handed versus right-handed computer mouse use: effect on upper-extremity posture. Y. Appl. Ergon. 2004, Jan. 35 (1):21–8.

DeRosa, E., Desmond, J., Anderson, A., Pfefferbaum, A., & Sullivan, E. The human basal forebrain integrates the old and the new. Neuron. 2004, Mar 4. 41(5):825–37.

Dirnberger, G., Duregger, C., Lindinger, G., & Lang, W. Habituation in a simple repetitive motor task: a study with movement related cortical potentials. Clin. Neurophysiol. 2004, Feb. 115 (2):378–84.

Eliassen, J., Baynes, K., & Gazzaniga, M. Anterior and posterior callosal contributions to simultaneous bimanual movements of the hands and fingers. 1: Brain. 2000, Dec.123 Pt 12:2501–11.

Falkiner, S., & Myers, S. When exactly can carpal tunnel syndrome be considered work-related? ANZ. J. Surg. 2002, Mar.72 (3):204–9.

Franz, E., Attentional distribution of task parameters to the two hands during bimanual performance of right and left handers. J. Mot. Behav. 2004, Mar.36 (1):71–81.

Franz, E., Rowse, A., & Ballantine, B. Does handedness determine which hand leads in a bimanual task? J. Mot. Behav. 2002, Dec.34 (4):409–14.

Gerloff, C., & Andres, F. Bimanual coordination and interhemispheric interaction. Acta. Psychol. (Amst). 2002, Jun.11 (2–3):161–86.

Gorynia, I., & Egenter, D. Intermanual coordination in relation to handedness, familial sinistrality and lateral preferences. Cortex. 2000, Feb. 36 (1):1–18.

Grafton, S., Hazeltine, E., & Ivry R.Motor sequence learning with the non dominant hand: A PET functional imaging study. Exp. Brain Res. 2002, Oct.146 (3):369–78.

Hager-Ross, C., & Schieber, M. Quantifying the independence of human finger movements: comparisons of digits, hands and movement frequencies. J. Neurosci. 2000, Nov. 15, 20 (22):8542–50.

Hall, S. Metacarpophalangeal flexion forces with respect to age, sex, and exercise habits. Med. Sci. Sports Exerc. 1981, 13 (5):329–31.

Hoffman, E., Chang, W., & Yim, K. Computer mouse operation: is the left handed user disadvantaged? Appl. Ergon. 1997, Aug. 28 (4):245–8.

Heuer, H. Blocking in rapid finger tapping: the role of variability in proximodistal coordination. Journal of Motor Behavior 6/1/1998.

Izquierdo, J., Garcia, M., Buxo, C., & Izquierdo, N. Factors leading to the Computer Vision Syndrome: an issue at the contemporary workplace. 1. Bol. Asoc. Med. P. R.2004, Mar-Apr. (92):103–10.

Jancke, L., Specht, K., Mirzazade, S., & Peters, M. The effect of finger movement speed of the dominant and the subdominant hand on cerebellar activation: a functional magnetic resonance imaging study. Neuroimage. 1999, May 9 (5):497–507.

Jensen C., Borg V., Finsen L., Hansen K., Juul-Kristensen B., Christensen H. Job demands, muscle activity and musculoskeletal symptoms in relation to work with the computer mouse. Scand J Work Environ Health. 1998, Oct; 24 (5):418–24.

Johnson P., Hagberg M., Hjelm E., Rempel D. Measuring and characterizing force exposures during computer mouse use. Scand J Work Environ Health. 2000, Oct; 26 (5):398–405.

Karlquist, L., Bernmark, E., Ekenvall, L., Hagberg, M., Isaksson, A., & Rosto, T. Computer mouse position as a determinant of posture, muscular load and perceived exertion. Scand. J. Work Environ. Health, 1998, Feb. 24 (1):62–73.

Karpitskaya, Y., Novak, C., & Mackinnon, S. Prevalence of smoking, obesity, diabetes mellitus, and thyroid disease in patients with carpal tunnel syndrome. Ann. Plast. Surg. 2002, Mar. 48 (3):269–73.

Keir, P., Bach, J., & Rempel, D. Effects of computer mouse design and task on carpal tunnel pressure. Ergonomics. 1999, Oct. 42 (10):1350–60.

Kimura, D, & Vanderwolf, C. The relation between hand preference and the performance of individual finger movements by left and right hand. Brain, 1970, 93, 769–774.

Klar, A. Human handedness and scalp hair-whorl direction develop from a common genetic mechanism. Genetics. 2003, Sep.165 (1):269–75.

Knecht S, Drager B, Deppe M, Bobe L, Lohmann H, Floel A, Ringelstein EB, & Henningsen H. Handedness and hemispheric language dominance in healthy humans. Brain. 2000, Dec; 123Pt 12:2512-8.

Henningsen, H. Handedness and hemispheric language dominance in healthy humans. Brain. 2000, Dec. 123 Pt 12:2512–8.

Kumar, S., & Mandal, M. Motor performance as a function of verbal, nonverbal interference and handedness. Int. J. Neurosci. 2004, Jul.114 (7):787–94.

Kurth, R., Villringer, K., Curio, G., Wolf, K., Krause, T., Repenthin, J., Schwieman, J., Deuchert, M., & Villringer, A. FMRI shows multiple somatotopic digit representations in human primary somatosensory cortex. Neuroreport. 2000, May 15. 11 (7):1487–91.

Kusack, J. The Light at the End of the Tunnel. ERIC EJ413629.1990-00-0.

Laursen, B., & Jensen, B. Shoulder muscle activity in young and older people during a computer mouse task. Clin Biomech. (Bristol, Avon). 2000, 15 Suppl. 1:S30-3.

Lee, K., Swanson, N., Sauter, S., Wickstrom, R., Waikar, A., & Mangum, M. A review of physical exercises recommended for VDT operators. Applied Ergonomics. 1992. 23 (6), 387–408.

Levy, J. Psychobiological Implication of Bilateral Asymmetry. Hemisphere Function in the Human Brain. Dimond & Beumont Editors, 1974, London: Paul Elek. Ltd.

Li, A., Yetkin, F., Cox, R., & Haughton, V. Ipsilateral hemisphere activation during motor and sensory tasks. AJNR Am. J. Neuroradiol. 1996, Apr.17 (4):651–5.

Lyall, J., Gliner, J., & Hubbell, M. Treatment of worker's compensation cases of carpal tunnel syndrome: an outcome study. J. Hand Ther. 2002, Jul.-Sep.15 (3):251–9.

Mack, L., Gonzalez, G., Tothi, L., & Heilman, K. Hemispheric specialization for handwriting in right handers. 1: Brain Cogn. 1993, Jan.21 (1):80–6.

Mani, L., & Gerr, F. Work-related upper extremity musculoskeletal disorders. Prim. Care. 2000, Dec.27 (4):845–64.

Mapp, A., Ono, H., & Barbeito, R. What does the dominant eye dominate? A brief and somewhat contentious review. Percept. Psychophys. 2003, Feb.65 (2):310–7.

McDiarmid, M., Oliver, M., Ruser, J., & Gucer, P. Male and female rate differences in carpal tunnel syndrome injuries: personal attributes or job tasks. Environ. Res. 2000, May 83 (1):23–32.

McManus, I., Kemp, R., & Grant, J. Differences between fingers and hands in tapping ability: dissociation between speed and regularity. Cortex, 1986, Sep.22 (3):461–73.

Mohr, C., Landis, T., Bracha, H.,, & Brugger, P. Opposite turning behavior in right handers and non right handers suggests a link between handedness and cerebral dopamine asymmetries. Behav. Neurosci. 2003, Dec.117 (6):1448–52.

Muggleton, J., Allen, R., & Chappell, P. Hand and arm injuries associated with repetitive manual work in industry: a review of disorders, risk factors and preventive measures. Ergonomics. 1999, 42, 714–739.

Muller, R., Kleinhans, N., Pierce, K., Kemmotsu, N., & Courchesne E. Brain Res. Cogn. Brain Res. 2002, Aug. 14 (2):277–93.

Nachshon, I. Directional preferences in perception of visual stimuli. Int. J. Neurosci. 1985, Jan.25 (3–4):161–74.

Nadler, M., Harrison, L., & Stephens, J. Acquisition of a new motor skill is accompanied by changes incutaneomuscular reflex responses recorded from finger muscles in man. Exp. Brain Res. 2000, Sep.134 (2):246–54.

Nakada, T., Fujii, Y., & Kwee, I. Coerced training of the non dominant hand resulting in cortical reorganization: a high-field functional magnetic resonance imaging study. J. Neurosurg. 2004, Aug.101 (2):310–3.

Nalcaci, E., Kalaycioglu, C., Cicek, M., & Gene, Y. The relationship between handedness and fine motor performance. Cortex. 2001, Sep.37 (4):493–500.

Nebes, R., Handedness and the perception of part whole relationships. Cortex. 1991, 7, 350–356.

Nord, S., Ettare, D., Drew, D., & Hodge, S. Muscle learning therapy-efficacy of a biofeedback based protocol in treating work related upper extremity disorders. J. Occup. Rehabil. 2001, Mar. 11 (1):23–31.

Ong, C., Chia, S., Jeyaratnam, J., & Tan, K.. Musculoskeletal disorders among operators of visual display terminals. Scan. J. Work Environ. Health. 1995, Feb.21 (1):60–4.

OSHA Ergonomic Solutions Computer Workstations eTool—Components-Keyboards. http://www.osha.gov .

Pascarelli, E., & Hsu, Y. Understanding work-related upper extremity disorders: clinical findings in 485 computer users, musicians, and others. J. Occup. Rehabil. 2001, Mar.11 (1):1–21.

Parlow, S., & Kinsbourne, M. Asymmetrical transfer of training between hands: implications for interhemispheric communication in normal brain. Brain and Cognition. 1989, Sep.11 (1):98–113.

Pascarelli, E., & Kella, J. Soft tissue injuries related to use of the computer keyboard. A clinical study of 53 severely injured persons. J. Occup. Med. 1993, May 35 (5):522–32.

Peter, M., & Ivanoff, J. Performance asymmetries in computer mouse control of right-handers, and left-handers with left and right handed mouse experience. Journal of Motor Behavior. 1999, 31, 86–94.

Rediff.com, Computer Related Injuries are on the rise, chances are, you may have them too, February 28, 2001.

Reiss, M., & Reiss, G. Motor asymmetry. Fortschr. Neurol. Psychiatr. 2000, Feb.68 (2):70–9.

Rigal, R. Which handedness: preference or performance? Percept. Mot. Skills. 1992, Dec.75 (3Pt 1):851–66.

Riss, W. Testing a theory of brain function by computer methods. Brain Behav. Evol. 1984, 24 (1):13–20.

Sadato, N., Yonekura, Y., Waki, A., Yamada, H, & Ishii Y. Role of the supplementary motor area and the right pre motor cortex in the coordination of bimanual finger movements. J. Neurosci. 1997, Dec. 15. 17(24):9667–74.

Satz, P. Pathological Left-Handedness: An Explanatory Model. Cortex 1972, June.

Sforza, C., Macri, C., Turci, M., Grassi, G., & Ferrario, V. Neuromuscular patterns of finger movements during piano playing: Definition of an experimental protocol. Ital. J. Anat. Embryol. 2003, Oct.-Dec. 108 (4) 211–22.

Siebner, H. Limmer, C., Peinemann, A., Drzezga, A., Bloem, B., Schwaiger, M., & Conrad B. Long-term consequences of switching handedness: a positron emission tomography study on handwriting in "converted" left-handers. J. Neurosci. 2002, Apr. 1; 22 (7):2816–25.

Solodkin, A., Hlustik, P., Noll, D., & Small, S. Lateralization of motor circuits and handedness during finger movements. Eur. J. Neurol. 2001, Sep. 8 (5):425–34.

Soros, P., Knecht, S., Imai, T., Gurtler, S., Lutkenhoner, B., Ringelstein, E.,B & Henningsen, H. Cortical asymmetries of the human somatosensory hand representation in right and left handers. Neurosci. Letters. 1999, Aug. 20; 271 (2):89–92.

Sproule, J., Tansey, C., Burns, B., & Fenelon, G. The Web: friend or foe of the hand surgeon? Hand Surg. 2003, Dec.8 (2):181–5.

Stancak, A. Jr., & Pfurtscheller, G. The effects of handedness and type of movement on the contralateral preponderance of mu rhythm desynchronisation. Electroencephalongr. Clin. Neurophysiol. 1996, Aug. 99 (2):174–82.

Stoeckel, M., Weder, B., Binkofski, F., Choi, H. Amunts, K., Pieperhoff, P., Shah, N., & Seitz, R. Left and right superior parietal lobule in tactile object discrimination. Eur. J. Neurosci. 2004, Feb.19 (4):1067–72.

Summers, J., Byblow, W., Bysouth-Youth, D. & Semjen, A. Bimanual circle drawing during secondary task loading. Motor Control. 1998, Apr.2 (2):106–13.

Tankle, R., & Heilman, K. Mirror writing in right-handers and in left-handers. 1: Brain. 1983, May 19(1):115–23.

Taniguchi. M., Yoshimine, T., Cheyne, D., Kato, A., Kihara, T., Ninomiya, H., Hirata, M., Hirabuki, N., Nakamura, H., & Hayakawa, T. Neuromagnetic fields preceding unilateral movements in dextrals and sinistrals. Neuroreport. 1998, May 11 9 (7):1497–502.

The John Marshall Journal of Computer & Information Law, Vol. X111 *Spring 1995* No.3. Repetitive stress injuries and the computer keyboard: Is there still no causal relationship between use and injury; is it wise to warn?

Travers, P., & Stanton, B. Office workers and video display terminals: physical, psychological and ergonomic factors. AAOHN J. 2002, Nov.50 (11):489–93.

Treffner, P., & Turvey, M.. Symmetry, broken symmetry and handedness in bimanual coordination dynamics. Exp. Brain Res. 1996,107 (3):463–78.

Ullen, F., & Bengtsson, S. Independent processing of the temporal and ordinal structure of movement sequences. J. Neurophysiol. 2003, Dec.90 (6):3725–35.

Whitall, Jill. Bimanual Finger tapping: effects of frequency and auditory information on timing consistency and coordination. J. of Motor Behavior, 6/1/2000.

Ubelacker, S. Teachers Parents! Beware of RSI. ERIC ED425002, 1998-12-00, p.6.

Vaid, J., Bellugi, U., & Poizner, H. Hand dominance for signing: clues to brain lateralization of language. Neurophsychologia. 1989, 27 (7):949–60.

Van Dijk, M., Reitsma, J., Fischer, J., & Sanders. G. Indications for requesting laboratory tests for concurrent diseases in patients with carpal tunnel syndrome: a systematic review. Clin. Chem. 2003, Sep. 49 (9):1437–44.

Wada, J. & Rasmussen, T. Intracarotid Injection of Sodium Amytol for the Lateralization of Speech Dominance. Neurosurgery. 1960. 17: 266–282.

Wessel, K., Zeffiro, T., Toro, C., & Hallett, M. Self paced versus metronome paced finger movements: At positron emission tomography study. J. Neuroimagine. 1997, Jul.7 (3):145–51.

Wilke, J., & Sheeley, E. Muscular or directional preferences in finger movement as a function of handedness. Cortex. 1979, Dec.15 (4):561–9.

Yu, I., & Wong, T. Musculoskeletal problems among VDU workers in a Hong Kong bank. Occup. Med. (Lond.). 1996, Aug. 46 (4):275–80.

## BOOKS

Bibliography. <u>Cumulative trauma disorders in the workplace,</u> CDC. NIOSH..
   Education and Information Division, 1995. Cincinnati, Ohio 45226.
Blau, T. <u>The Psychological Examination of the Child</u>. 1991, Wiley Publishers.
Bragdon, A., & Gamon, D. <u>Brains that work a little bit differently.</u> 2000,
   Barnes and Nobles Publishers.
Coren, S. <u>The Left Handers Syndrome.</u> 1992, The Free Press. 866 Third Ave.,
   NY. NY. 10022.
Dent, G. <u>Return to Work...by Design.</u> 1990, Martin-Dennison Press, Stock-
   ton, Ca.
Edwards, B. <u>Drawing on the Right Side of the Brain</u>. 1983, Amazon.com
Grafton, C. <u>Tennis: Starting Off Right or Left.</u> 1980, Winning Ways, Okla.
   City, Okla.
Klafs, C. & Arnheim, D. <u>Modern Principles of Athletic Training</u>. 1973, St.
   Louis: C. V. Mosby.
Lauckner, K. & Lintner, M. <u>The Computer Continuum.</u> Second Edition.
   Prentice Hall, Upper Saddle River, New Jersey 07458.
Newell, J. <u>Using Case Management to Improve Health Outcomes</u>. 1996,
   <u>Aspen Publishers</u>, Gaethersberg, Md.
Reed, P. <u>The Medical Disability Advisor.</u> Reed Group, Inc. 1997, Boulder,
   Colo. 80302.
Smith, A, <u>The Mind.</u> 1984, The Viking Press, 40 West 23rd Street, NY, NY ,
   10010.
Springer, S. & Deutsch, G. <u>Left Brain, Right Brain.</u> 1989, W. H. Freeman,
   N.Y. N.Y.
Trembley, D. <u>Learning to use your Aptitudes</u>. 1974. San Louis Obispo: Erin
   Hills Publishers.

LaVergne, TN USA
16 August 2010
193479LV00003B/66/P